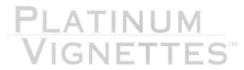

PLATINUM
VIGNETTES™

ULTRA-HIGH-YIELD CLINICAL CASE SCENARIOS
FOR USMLE STEP 2

Obstetrics &
Gynecology

PLATINUM VIGNETTES™

ULTRA-HIGH-YIELD CLINICAL CASE SCENARIOS
FOR USMLE STEP 2

Obstetrics & Gynecology

ADAM BROCHERT, MD

Resident
Department of Radiology
Medical College of Georgia
Memorial Health University Medical Center
Savannah, Georgia

Hanley & Belfus, Inc. / Philadelphia

Publisher: HANLEY & BELFUS, INC.
Medical Publishers
210 South 13th Street
Philadelphia, PA 19107
(215) 546-7293; 800-962-1892
FAX (215) 790-9330
Web site: http://www.hanleyandbelfus.com

Note to the reader: Although the information in this book has been carefully reviewed for correctness of dosage and indications, neither the author nor the publisher can accept any legal responsibility for any errors or omissions that may be made. Neither the publisher nor the author makes any warranty, expressed or implied, with respect to the material contained herein. Before prescribing any drug, the reader must review the manufacturer's current product information (package inserts) for accepted indications, absolute dosage recommendations, and other information pertinent to the safe and effective use of the product described. This is especially important when drugs are given in combination or as an adjunct to other forms of therapy.

PLATINUM VIGNETTES™: OBSTETRICS & GYNECOLOGY   ISBN 1-56053-532-6

Library of Congress Control Number: 2002102752

Last digit is the print number: 9 8 7 6 5 4 3 2 1

INTRODUCTION

Case scenarios are a great way to review for the USMLE Step 2 exam. A high percentage of current exam questions center on case studies or patient presentations in an office or emergency department setting. Practicing this format and being familiar with the majority of the classic, "guaranteed-to-be-on-the-exam" case scenarios gives the examinee an obvious, clear-cut advantage. *Platinum Vignettes*™ were written to offer you that advantage.

You need to be familiar not only with pathophysiology, but also the work-up and management of several conditions to succeed on the USMLE Step 2 exam. Sifting through the history, physical exam findings, and various tests, you are expected to make and confirm the diagnosis and manage the patient's condition.

Each book in the *Platinum Vignettes*™ presents 50 case scenarios or clinical vignettes. The individual vignettes are followed by the diagnosis, pathophysiology, diagnostic strategies, and management issues pertaining to that specific patient. The reader must turn the page to obtain these latter details, and is encouraged to "guess" before reading about the patient's condition and course. In fact, you are advised not only to guess the diagnosis, but also to postulate on which test to order next, what therapy to give, and what to "watch out" for in the condition presented.

Important words or phrases ("buzzwords") are set in bold type in the explanation of each vignette. These words or phrases indicate the material most commonly asked about on the exam or are important in helping to distinguish one condition from another. This format is designed for review of material that was previously learned during rotations; therefore, further reading is advised if the topic or buzzwords are unfamiliar. Remember, buzzwords are rarely helpful unless you know what they mean!

Every attempt was made to provide the most current, up-to-date information on every topic tackled in this volume and every volume in the series—but medicine is a rapidly changing field. If you hear about a new therapy in a conference or on rounds, it may well be that the standard of care has changed. Remember, though, that what you see on the wards and in the office isn't always applicable to the boards (e.g., everyone with pneumonia should not be given the latest "big-gun" antibiotic; all patients with headaches should not receive a CT scan).

Good luck!

ADAM BROCHERT, MD

NOTE: A standard Table of Contents, with cases listed by diagnosis, would give you too much of a head start on solving each patient scenario. Challenge yourself! When ready, you can turn to the detailed Case Index at the back of this book.

Gynecology

History

A 20-year-old woman comes into the office complaining of pain during urination, increased frequency of urination, and a yellowish vaginal discharge for the past 3 days. She thinks she may have a yeast infection, which she is prone to developing, and asks for an antifungal drug prescription. The patient denies additional symptoms and has no other significant past medical history. Her only medication is oral contraceptives. She mentions an allergy to ampicillin, which gave her a rash several years ago.

The patient uses marijuana and cocaine on the weekends and likes to drink alcohol 3–4 times per week. She is sexually active with multiple partners.

Exam

T: 98.9°F   BP: 118/76   RR: 14/min. P: 64/min.

The patient is athletic appearing and is in no acute distress. Head, neck, chest, abdominal, and extremity exams are unremarkable. Pelvic examination reveals a yellowish, thin, purulent cervical discharge. Her cervix is also reddened and somewhat friable. A swab of the discharge is placed on a slide and viewed under a microscope (see figure).

Tests

Hemoglobin: 14 g/dL (normal 12–16)
White blood cell (WBC) count: 9900/μL (normal 4500–11,000)
AST: 22 u/L (normal 7–27)

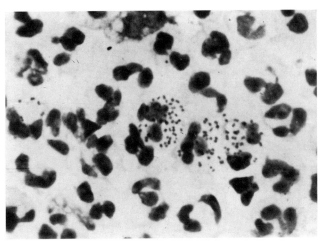

intracellular
diplococci of NG

From Cunha BA: Infectious Disease Pearls. Philadelphia, Hanley & Belfus, Inc., 1999, p 3.

Cervicitis secondary to *Neisseria gonorrhoeae* infection

The photo shows the classic appearance of intracellular diplococci inside **white blood cells.** The diplococci are gram negative and appear red in color photos.

Pathophysiology

Gonorrhea is spread by sexual contact and therefore can be seen in the vagina/cervix, **rectum, pharynx,** and, occasionally, the **eyes.** In the female pelvis, gonorrhea can lead to the development of pelvic inflammatory disease (PID). It can also occasionally disseminate hematogenously to the **skin, joints, perihepatic region,** and other areas.

Diagnosis & Treatment

Though gonorrhea can be asymptomatic, classic symptoms include **vaginal discharge, dysuria/painful urination,** and **urinary frequency.** Classic presentation includes a history of being sexually active with **multiple partners** or a partner with risk factors (i.e., **drug user, promiscuous**). Note that some patients may be embarrassed about this behavior, and deny it.

On exam of the vagina and/or cervix, the discharge is often seen. It is typically **yellowish or whitish** and **mucopurulent** (a combination of pus-like and mucus-like). The cervix is inflamed and may be **reddened** and/or **friable.** A gram stain of the discharge classically reveals **intracellular** (within WBCs) **gram-negative diplococci,** allowing a presumptive diagnosis to be made before culture results are available. **Culture** is the **gold standard** for diagnosis, however.

Treatment regimens must cover gonorrhea *and* chlamydia (coinfection is presumed in the setting of gonorrhea, though the reverse is not always true because gonorrhea is usually easier to detect). Gonorrhea can be treated with a **single dose** (good for noncompliant patients) of **intramuscular ceftriaxone** (*safe* in pregnancy). Ciprofloxacin or ofloxacin are other alternate single-dose oral regimens, but both should be *avoided* in pregnancy. A **single oral dose** of **azithromycin** can treat chlamydia, as can a 1-week regimen of **doxycycline,** ofloxacin, or **erythromycin** (the treatment of choice in pregnancy, though amoxicillin is an alternative).

Standard treatment includes identifying and treating all **sexual partners.**

More High-Yield Facts

Screen asymptomatic, sexually active women **under age 25** every 6–12 months for gonorrhea/chlamydia with cultures (to prevent PID/infertility).

Gonorrhea is the **most common cause** of **septic arthritis** in younger, sexually active adults.

Case 2
Gynecology

History

A 21-year-old woman is experiencing irregular menstrual periods with intermittent, mild-to-moderate lower abdominal pain and cramping. She says that lately her periods are occurring very infrequently and that she has only had two in the last 12 months. However, the patient also mentions that her periods have always been somewhat irregular and less frequent than her peers. She has been trying to get pregnant, unsuccessfully, for the past 2 years. When her periods do come, they are often heavy, requiring 8 to 10 pads per day for 3 to 4 days.

Exam

T: 98.5°F   BP: 138/88   RR: 16/min.   P: 74/min.

The patient is obese and has excessive facial hair in a male-pattern distribution. She also has some mild facial acne. Breast and genitalia exams are unremarkable. Pelvic exam reveals slight smooth enlargement of both ovaries with no masses palpated. No other abnormalities are identified.

Tests

Hemoglobin: 13 g/dL (normal 12–16)
White blood cell count: 6800/μL (normal 4500–11,000)
Fasting glucose level: 120 mg/dL
   (normal fasting 70–110)
Thyroid-stimulating hormone (TSH):
   2.3 μU/mL (normal 0.5–5)
Prolactin level: 5 ng/mL (normal 2–15)
Luteinizing hormone (LH):follicle-
   stimulating hormone (FSH) ratio = 4:1
Free testosterone level: 2.3 ng/dL
   (normal 0.1–1.3)
Dehydroepiandrosterone (DHEA) level:
   10 ng/mL (normal 1.4–8.0)

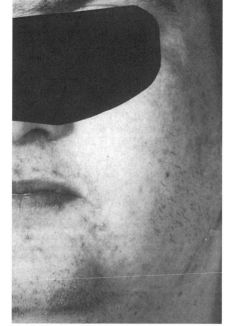

From Becker KL, et al (eds): Principles and Practice of Endocrinology and Metabolism. Philadelphia, Lippincott, 1990, pp 834–848; with permission.

Polycystic ovary syndrome (Stein-Leventhal syndrome)

The picture shows hirsutism.

Pathophysiology

Polycystic ovary syndrome (PCO) is **idiopathic,** but is a common, benign disorder. Clinical findings are thought to result from a hormonal imbalance, with a **high LH level,** which causes suppression of FSH secretion and results in a **high LH:FSH ratio (> 2:1).** This imbalance then leads to increased androgen secretion and **high androgen levels** (high levels of **testosterone, androstenedione,** and **DHEA**), which are converted to estrogen and also result in **increased estrogen levels.** Many affected patients are also prone to **insulin resistance.**

Diagnosis & Treatment

Classic clinical findings include **hirsutism, oligo- or amenorrhea, infertility,** and **obesity.** Additionally, most women are under age 30 at first presentation. Mild **hyperglycemia/insulin resistance** is also fairly common, and patients are at an increased risk for type II diabetes. Most women have a **long history** of menstrual irregularities and hirsutism, beginning around the time of menarche.

The clinical diagnosis can be clinched if an **elevated LH level** (or increased LH:FSH ratio) is present in a woman who **has bleeding after receiving progesterone** (indicating estrogen is present) in the standard work-up for amenorrhea. Increased androgen levels are also present.

Treatment includes **weight loss** for those who are obese (about 50% of affected patients) and "forced" menses to prevent **endometrial hyperplasia** (and the **increased risk of endometrial carcinoma**) due to **unopposed estrogen stimulation.** This is usually done with **oral contraceptive pills,** but a progestational agent can also be given for 10 days each month. Women who desire to become pregnant can often do so with **clomiphene.**

More High-Yield Facts

Make sure there is not a **prolactinoma** (high prolactin levels, bilateral nipple discharge) or **hypothyroidism** (high TSH level, other hypothyroid symptoms) as a cause of menstrual irregularities.

Estrogen-secreting neoplasms are a very rare cause of PCO-type symptoms. The history will mention fairly **recent or quick onset** of symptoms in an **older** woman. Classically, an ovarian mass will be present on physical exam or by ultrasound.

Always check the human chorionic gonadotropin level first to rule out pregnancy in any case of amenorrhea.

Case 3

Gynecology

History

A 55-year-old woman is troubled by urinary incontinence. She says she involuntarily loses urine after coughing, sneezing, or straining, and while jogging. Symptoms have gradually worsened over the last 3 years, beginning shortly after her menopause began. The patient also mentions a feeling of pelvic "heaviness" that is aggravated by prolonged standing and relieved by lying down. She has 6 children, all delivered vaginally without complications. She does not smoke, and her only medication is acetaminophen for arthritis in her left knee.

Exam

T: 98.2°F   BP: 128/84   RR: 14/min.   P: 78/min.

The patient appears healthy and is in no acute distress. Breast and abdominal exams are unremarkable. No ovarian masses are appreciated on pelvic exam. When the patient is asked to bear down, a bulge can be felt along the upper anterior vaginal wall. When she is asked to cough, a short spurt of urine escapes the urethra.

Tests

Hemoglobin: 14 g/dL (normal 12–16)
White blood cell count: 7000/μL (normal 4500–11,000)
Urinalysis: negative for glucose, protein, bacteria, white blood cells, and red blood cells; normal specific gravity

Stress incontinence

This disorder is often secondary to uterine prolapse and cystocele formation (as in the present patient).

Pathophysiology

Stress incontinence is a common complaint in women after menopause, especially those who have had multiple vaginal deliveries. The supporting ligaments of the pelvic organs can be **weakened** by repeated deliveries, and they can also **atrophy** somewhat after menopause, especially in women who do not take hormone replacement. This is sometimes called "pelvic relaxation."

Pelvic relaxation can cause bulging of pelvic organs into the vagina (**vaginal prolapse**), often in the form of cystocele, rectocele, and/or urethrocele formation (see below). In the case of a cystocele, the bladder bulges into the upper anterior wall of the vagina. The lowering of the bladder neck and proximal urethra allows any increase in intra-abdominal pressure to be transmitted to the bladder, which **overcomes urethral resistance** and causes involuntary loss of urine.

Diagnosis & Treatment

The classic history for stress incontinence is **involuntary urine loss after coughing, sneezing, straining, or exercising** (activities that cause **increased intra-abdominal pressure**). Urinary **frequency** and **urgency** may also occur. Many patients complain of **pelvic heaviness or fullness,** typically **aggravated by prolonged standing** and **relieved by lying down.** Most affected patients are **postmenopausal** and multiparous (**multiple vaginal deliveries**).

On examination, a **bulge can be felt in the upper anterior vaginal wall** and **involuntary urine loss** may occur when the patient bears down. The **"Q-tip test"** can be used to confirm the diagnosis. A Q-tip is inserted into the urethra and the patient is asked to bear down. In stress incontinence, the Q-tip angle increases beyond normal limits during straining.

Initial (conservative) treatment includes **pelvic strengthening** (e.g., Kegel) **exercises,** a **pessary** (artificial physical support device inserted into the vagina), and **avoidance** of activities that increase intra-abdominal pressure. Patients may also want to wear **protective undergarments. Estrogen** replacement therapy may help delay or improve symptoms. **Surgery** is reserved for severe cases and those that fail conservative management.

More High-Yield Facts

Other types of prolapse: **Rectoceles** cause **trouble defecating**; the rectum bulges into the **lower posterior** vaginal wall. **Urethroceles** cause urinary incontinence; the urethra bulges into the **lower anterior** vaginal wall. **Enteroceles** cause few specific symptoms; loops of bowel bulge into the **upper posterior** vaginal wall.

Gynecology

History

A 31-year-old woman has made an appointment because she is concerned about vaginal discharge. She says the discharge began several days ago and is heavy, light green–colored, and foul smelling. Additional symptoms include urinary frequency, vaginal itching and burning, and pain during sexual intercourse. The woman has two current sexual partners and uses no birth control. She drinks alcohol, but denies smoking or drug use and is currently taking no medications.

Exam

T: 98.3°F   BP: 118/76   RR: 12/min.   P: 70/min.

The patient appears healthy and is in no acute distress. Breast and abdominal exams are unremarkable. Speculum exam reveals a fairly profuse, thin, frothy discharge that is yellow-green and malodorous. Vaginal erythema and multiple cervical petechiae, giving the cervix a "strawberry" appearance, are also present. A wet-smear of the discharge reveals a motile organism (see figure) and white blood cells. A potassium hydroxide preparation is negative.

Tests

Hemoglobin: 14 g/dL (normal 12–16)
White blood cell (WBC) count: 7000/μL (normal 4500–11,000)
Urinalysis: negative for glucose, protein, bacteria, WBCs, and RBCs; normal
    specific gravity

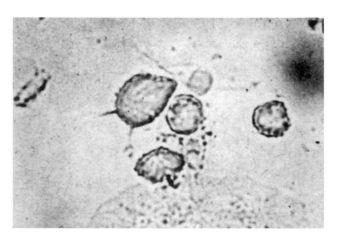

From Eschenbach DA. In Scott JR, et al (eds): Danforth's Obstetrics and Gynecology, 7th ed. Philadelphia, Lippincott, 1988, pp 641–664; with permission.

Pathophysiology

T. vaginalis is a **sexually transmitted, motile** protozoa with multiple **flagella** that has the ability to adhere to epithelial cells. It can be *asymptomatic,* especially in *males.* The organism produces gas bubbles (creating the frothy appearance of the discharge) and causes a discharge with an **elevated pH (> 4.5).**

Diagnosis & Treatment

Classic symptoms include a **profuse, malodorous, frothy, and greenish-gray discharge** as well as **vaginal itching, burning,** and **discomfort. Dyspareunia** and **dysuria** are also common. Patients are often **promiscuous** and rarely use condoms. Those who seek delayed treatment often describe a **worsening of symptoms shortly after menses** (thought to be due to pH changes that favor the organism).

Physical exam reveals **erythema** and **edema** of the **vagina** and a "**strawberry cervix,**" which describes multiple **petechiae** on an **inflamed-appearing cervix.** A wet (i.e. saline) smear of the discharge reveals the organism. Culture is the gold standard for diagnosis, but it is not needed if the organism is visualized directly.

Treatment is **metronidazole,** given either as a large single dose (noncompliant patients; causes stomach upset in many) or over 7 days. Remember that patients must **avoid alcohol** while taking metronidazole (causes a disulfiram-like reaction), and the drug is a **teratogen** (delay treatment until after the first trimester during pregnancy).

More High-Yield Facts

Don't forget to **treat sexual partners,** even if they are asymptomatic.

Trichomonas and other causes of vaginitis can *interfere* with Pap smear results. Treat the infection and **repeat the Pap smear** in a few months in this setting.

Case 5
Gynecology

History

A 59-year-old woman presents with a chief complaint of constipation plus abdominal and pelvic swelling and fullness. She mentions that she began feeling a vague sensation of pelvic fullness, bloating, and mild constipation a few months ago. Eventually, she noticed abdominal swelling as well. The patient involuntarily lost 20 pounds over the last 2 months and has been experiencing anorexia. She is nulliparous and went through menopause 1 year ago. She has a family history of breast and ovarian cancer, but had a negative screening mammogram 1 year ago. She takes no medications.

Exam

T: 98.3°F   BP: 128/84   RR: 16/min.   P: 82/min.

The patient is in no acute distress. Her sclerae are pale. Breast, lung, and cardiac exams are unremarkable. Abdominal exam reveals bulging flanks, a positive fluid wave, and shifting dullness to percussion. Bowel sounds are normal, and no masses are appreciated. Pelvic exam reveals a solid, irregular, fixed pelvic mass on the left.

Tests

Hemoglobin: 10 g/dL (normal 12–16)
Ferritin: 340 µg/L (normal 20–200)
White blood cell count: 7000/µL (normal 4500–11,000)
CA-125 level: 98 kU/mL (normal < 35)
Urinalysis: negative for glucose, protein, bacteria, white blood cells, and red blood cells; normal specific gravity

Pathophysiology

Risk factors for ovarian cancer include **age** (average age at presentation is **60**), **nulliparity** (or advanced age at time of first pregnancy), **early menarche, late menopause,** and a **positive family history** of **breast** or **ovarian** cancer. Ovarian cancer is the **leading cause of death from gynecologic cancer** and the **fourth overall** cause of cancer death in women.

Most ovarian cancers are **epithelial** in origin (e.g., **serous** and **mucinous** adeno-carcinomas), as opposed to **germ cell** (e.g., teratoma, yolk sac tumor) or **stromal** (e.g., fibroma) origin. The most common type is **serous cystadenocarcinoma,** which may feature **psammoma bodies** histologically.

Diagnosis & Treatment

Symptoms often don't occur until the tumor has spread **beyond the pelvis.** Vague abdominal complaints, such as **constipation, abdominal or pelvic "fullness,"** nausea, bloating, and **anorexia** are classic. **Abdominal swelling or distension** are often ominous signs, and may be related to ascites or tumor mass. Unintentional **weight loss** is also common. Patients sometimes present with findings of **large bowel obstruction.**

Physical exam may reveal **cachexia, ascites,** and a **pelvic/adnexal/ovarian mass** (classically **solid, irregular,** and/or **fixed**) or unilateral **ovarian enlargement.** Symptoms/signs of distant metastases may also be present. **Anemia** of chronic disease and an **elevated CA-125 level** (> 65 is fairly specific for ovarian cancer; false positives are common with lower levels) are also common. **Ultrasound** is often used as the initial imaging exam to characterize pelvic or ovarian masses, which are generally more solid than cystic if malignant.

Treatment involves **hysterectomy and bilateral salpingo-oophorectomy,** with surgical removal of any other visible tumor (**"debulking"**), which is usually in the **omentum/ peritoneal cavity** and **intra-abdominal lymph nodes.** Radiation and chemotherapy (regimen usually includes a **platinum-based agent** such as cisplatinum) are frequently used adjunctive measures. The 5-year survival is less than 25%, primarily due to late stage at presentation. Patients often die of complications from **bowel obstruction.**

More High-Yield Facts

Oral contraceptive pills **reduce the risk of ovarian cancer** by 50%.

Ovarian enlargement or an ovarian mass in a **postmenopausal** female is cancer *"until proven otherwise."*

Case 6

Gynecology

History

A 39-year-old black woman is experiencing painful and heavy periods, pelvic "pressure," bloating, and fatigue. She also mentions urinary frequency and some shortness of breath with exertion. All of these symptoms began gradually and have been getting steadily worse over the last several months. She denies depression, weight loss, and change in appetite, though she does mention craving ice cubes lately. The patient takes no medications and is otherwise in good health.

Exam

T: 98.7°F   BP: 130/88   RR: 18/min.   P: 92/min.

The patient is in no acute distress, but has mild tachypnea. Her sclerae and mucous membranes are pale. Breast, lung, cardiac, and abdominal exams are normal, with no tenderness to palpation in the abdomen. Pelvic exam reveals an enlarged, bulky, nontender uterus with several rounded, smooth protrusions. Her ovaries are not palpable because of the uterine size. Her cervix and vagina are normal. Stool is negative for occult blood.

Tests

Hemoglobin: 8 g/dL (normal 12–16)   WBCs: 7000/μL (4500–11,000)
Sodium: 139 meq/L (normal 135–145)   Creatinine: 1 mg/dL (normal 0.6–1.5)
Urinalysis: negative for glucose, protein, bacteria, WBCs, and RBCs; normal
    specific gravity
Peripheral blood smear: see figure
Abdominal x-ray: see figure

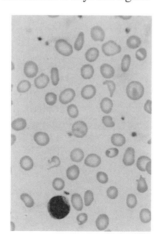

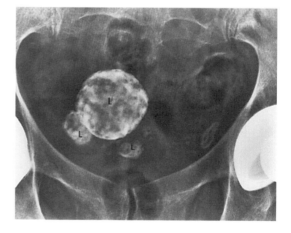

From Wood ME: Hematology/Oncology Secrets, 2nd ed. Color panels. Philadelphia, Hanley & Belfus, Inc., 1999; with permission.

From Katz DS, Math KR, Groskin SA (eds): Radiology Secrets. Philadelphia, Hanley & Belfus, Inc., 1998, pp 245–256; with permission.

Fibroid uterus with resultant dysmenorrhea and menorrhagia

The first figure shows the characteristic **hypochromic, microcytic RBCs** seen in iron-deficiency anemia. The second figure shows the typical appearance of **calcified fibroids** within three leimyomas (*L*).

Pathophysiology

Uterine leiomyomas ("**fibroids**") are the **most common benign tumor in women,** with roughly 20% of all women affected by age 40. They are seen more frequently and grow to a larger size in **black** women, and are **estrogen-dependent** tumors (may grow rapidly during pregnancy or estrogen use and often regress during menopause). Malignant degeneration is *extremely uncommon* (< 0.1%).

The tumors may either be **submucosal** (near the endometrium; may present as a pedunculated polyp protruding through the cervix), **intramural** (most common), or **subserosal** (near outer uterine wall).

Diagnosis & Treatment

Symptoms can vary widely, but classically include **pelvic pressure, heaviness or fullness, bloating, menorrhagia, dysmenorrhea,** and/or **urinary frequency** (from the tumor pushing on the bladder). Some fibroids may result in intermenstrual spotting (usually submucosal) or **infertility** (intramural tumors interfere with fetal growth and submucosal tumors can interfere with implantation).

Physical exam classically reveals an **enlarged, bulky, nontender uterus with several rounded, smooth protrusions.** The ovaries may not be palpable because of the enlarged uterus. Signs of **anemia** are common.

Pelvic **ultrasound** is generally the initial imaging test of choice to confirm the diagnosis and help rule out adnexal masses or other uterine pathology. Treatment is **observation** in most cases. Indications for treatment include excessive uterine bleeding that causes **anemia, large size** or **rapid growth,** severe **pelvic pain** or **dysmenorrhea, urinary symptoms** (frequency or retention), growth after menopause, and **infertility.** Treatment is usually **surgical/hysterectomy,** though **GnRH-agonists** can shrink the tumors, and a **myomectomy** can be tried for those who desire fertility.

More High-Yield Facts

Fibroids are the **most common indication** for **hysterectomy** and major abdominal surgery in women. They are also a common cause of pregnancy complications and indication for c-section due to rapid growth or location.

Women over age 35 with abnormal bleeding need a **dilatation and curettage** to rule out **endometrial carcinoma.**

Case 7

Gynecology

History

A 51-year-old woman comes into your office complaining of irritability and occasional, intense episodes of warmth, during which she flushes and then breaks out in a cold sweat. She also mentions insomnia and less frequent and increasingly irregular menstruation. Further questioning reveals a loss of interest in sex secondary to pain during intercourse, increasing vaginal burning, and urinary frequency and urgency. She denies depression and weight loss, and takes no regular medications.

Exam

T: 98.5°F   BP: 124/78   RR: 12/min.   P: 72/min.

The patient is in no acute distress and appears healthy. Breast, heart, lung, abdominal, and extremity exams are unremarkable. No skin lesions are identified. Pelvic examination reveals no masses. The lubricated speculum exam is painful for the patient. Her vaginal mucosa is smooth, dry, and somewhat whitish and irritated. A small focus of bleeding is caused by the speculum. The labia appear atrophic. Smear of a minimal vaginal discharge reveals a pH of 6, few epithelial cells, an increased number of parabasal cells, no pathologic bacteria, and a moderate number of white blood cells.

Tests

Hemoglobin: 14 g/dL (normal 12–16)
White blood cell (WBC) count: 7600/μL (normal 4500–11,000)
Sodium: 139 meq/L (normal 135–145)
Creatinine: 1 mg/dL (normal 0.6–1.5)
AST: 12 u/L (normal 7–27)
Luteinizing hormone (LH) level: 130 mU/mL (normal 2.5–40)
Follicle-stimulating hormone (FSH) level: 146 mU/mL (normal 5–40)
Estradiol: 20 pg/mL (normal 30–360)
Urinalysis: negative for glucose, protein, and bacteria; normal specific gravity

Pathophysiology

Menopause is the cessation of menses caused by natural ovarian failure and egg depletion, though it may also occur with surgical **ovarian removal** or **chemotherapy,** or due to **autoimmune** causes. It results in a deficiency of sex hormones (estrogen, progesterone, and testosterone) and elevated LH and FSH levels, which are the body's attempt to stimulate ovaries that are unable to respond. The average age of menopause in the U.S. is about **51.**

The loss of estrogen is associated with an **increased risk** of multiple conditions, including **osteoporosis, atherosclerotic cardiovascular disease,** and **cancer.** It also results in **atrophy of estrogen-responsive tissues,** such as glandular breast tissue, endometrium, pelvic supporting tissues, vaginal mucosa, and bladder. Some of these changes result in common menopausal symptoms (see below).

Diagnosis & Treatment

Classic symptoms include **oligo- or amenorrhea, hot flashes, sweats, irritability, emotional lability, insomnia, palpitations, dizziness, and fatigue.** Secondary symptoms such as **dyspareunia,** vaginal **burning,** vaginal mucosal irritability and friability, **urinary frequency,** and **dysuria** are due to atrophy of the genital and urinary tracts (atrophic vaginitis and urethritis). Pelvic relaxation may aggravate these genitourinary symptoms.

Physical exam is often normal. Changes of **atrophic vaginitis** include **dry, smooth, pale or whitish, and irritated vaginal mucosa.** There may be a scanty vaginal discharge that classically reveals **decreased epithelial cells, increased parabasal cells** (rounded epithelial cells), no pathologic bacteria, moderate WBCs, and an **increased pH** (> 5). Laboratory exam reveals **increased LH and FSH** and **decreased estradiol.**

Estrogen-replacement therapy promptly reduces general symptoms and those related to the genitourinary tract. It also lowers the risk of cardiovascular disease and osteoporosis, but increases the risk of endometrial cancer if progesterone is not given. Most physicians (supported by the scientific literature) believe the benefits of therapy outweigh the risks. Every woman must make her own decision after weighing the risks and benefits. Local **topical estrogens** can be used to reduce genitourinary symptoms in women who do not want the systemic effects of estrogen.

More High-Yield Facts

Postmenopausal women who smoke *can* receive hormone replacement therapy (but premenopausal female smokers *shouldn't* be given oral contraceptive pills due to the increased risk of thromboembolic disease).

Gynecology

History

A 29-year-old woman presents with multiple problems that seem to occur in the week before menstruation every month, then get better a few days after her period starts. Her symptoms include irritability, mood swings, trouble concentrating, fatigue, breast tenderness, cramping, headaches, and bloating. She says the symptoms have been going on for 3–4 years and occur every month "like clockwork," but are getting worse.

Recently, the symptoms have become bad enough that her ability to work is impaired and she has had to call in sick several times. She says her headaches, cramping, and breast tenderness respond to aspirin, but the other symptoms do not. She has never been pregnant and describes "normal" menstrual flow for roughly 4 days each month and regular, predictable cycles. The patient has no medical or psychiatric history and is otherwise in good health. She does not smoke, drink alcohol, or use other drugs.

Exam

T: 98.6°F   BP: 116/70   RR: 12/min.   P: 66/min.

The patient appears healthy, but is somewhat irritable. The sclerae are anicteric. Heart, lung, abdominal, and extremity exams are unremarkable. Her breasts are tender to palpation bilaterally, but no masses are appreciated. No skin lesions are identified. Pelvic examination is normal.

Tests

Hemoglobin: 14 g/dL (normal 12–16)
White blood cell count: 6500/μL (normal 4500–11,000)
Sodium: 139 meq/L (normal 135–145)
Creatinine: 1 mg/dL (normal 0.6–1.5)
AST: 12 u/L (normal 7–27)
Glucose: 80 mg/dL (normal fasting 70–110 mg/dL)
Urinalysis: negative for glucose, protein, and bacteria; normal specific gravity

Premenstrual dysphoric disorder (PMDD)

PMDD is a severe form of **premenstrual syndrome.**

Pathophysiology

Many women experience symptoms, including breast tenderness, fatigue, cramping, and bloating, in the days preceding menstrual flow. When symptoms become severe enough to interfere with work, school, or social activities, PMDD is said to be present. It is estimated that roughly **5% of women** are affected at some point during their reproductive years. The etiology is **unknown,** and no specific hormonal imbalance has been shown, though by definition the disorder is related to the menstrual cycle.

Diagnosis & Treatment

Symptoms include **irritability, tension, depressed mood, mood swings, decreased interest in usual activities, difficulty concentrating, lethargy, marked change in appetite, insomnia or hypersomnia, a sense of being overwhelmed,** and physical symptoms such as **breast tenderness, headaches, cramping, and bloating.**

There are formal diagnostic criteria that serve as a guide for recognizing the disorder; they need not be memorized. To formally diagnose PMDD, five or more of the above symptoms (including at least one "emotional" symptom) must occur during the week or two before the menstrual period (the luteal phase) and **remit a few days after the onset of menstruation** during most cycles in the past year. The symptoms must significantly **interfere with everyday activities or relationships** and cannot be an exacerbation of another disorder (e.g., depression). *Symptoms should be absent at other times during the menstrual cycle.*

The only FDA-approved treatment is **fluoxetine** (though using other serotonin-specific reuptake inhibitors is reasonable). **Aspirin/NSAIDs** are helpful for physical symptoms only. Many other treatments have been tried, but **none are proven to work** (e.g., vitamins, no sweets or caffeine, birth control pills, danazol, progesterone). Certain drugs may help with certain symptoms (e.g., benzodiazepines for anxiety, spironolactone for fluid retention). **GnRH-agonists** can eliminate symptoms, but induce a "medical menopause" with its own set of symptoms and health risks.

More High-Yield Facts

Affected women have an **increased risk of depression,** which can be aggravated by the luteal phase. Other disorders, such as **migraine headaches** and asthma, may also be affected by the luteal phase.

Gynecology

History

A 17-year-old girl is concerned because she has never had a period and has not developed breasts like most of her peers. She wonders if there is something wrong with her. She is otherwise in good health and currently takes no medications. Past surgical history is remarkable for neck surgery as an infant for "some type of tumor." The patient does not smoke or use drugs and denies frequent, strenuous exercise or concerns about her weight.

Exam

T: 98.7°F   BP: 126/74   RR: 14/min.   P: 68/min.

The patient is short in stature. She has slight webbing of her neck, which is short, and a low posterior hairline, along with a well-healed surgical scar in the left supraclavicular area. Chest examination reveals a broad chest with broadly spaced nipples and a complete lack of breast development (see figure). Axillary hair has not developed. The patient has an abnormally increased carrying angle at the elbow. Abdominal exam is unremarkable. The genitalia are prepubescent in appearance, with a lack of adult-type pubic hair. Pelvic exam reveals the presence of a cervix and uterus, but the ovaries cannot be palpated.

Tests

Hemoglobin: 15 g/dL (normal 12–16)
White blood cell count: 6500/μL (normal 4500–11,000)
Sodium: 139 meq/L (normal 135–145)
Creatinine: 1 mg/dL (normal 0.6–1.5)
AST: 12 u/L (normal 7–27)
Glucose: 80 mg/dL (normal fasting 70–110 mg/dL)
Luteinizing hormone level: 122 mU/mL (normal 2.5–40)
Follicle-stimulating hormone level: 136 mU/mL (normal 5–40)
Estradiol: 18 pg/mL (normal 30–360)
Urinalysis: negative for glucose, protein, and bacteria; normal specific gravity
Buccal smear: normal-appearing epithelial cells, no Barr bodies identified

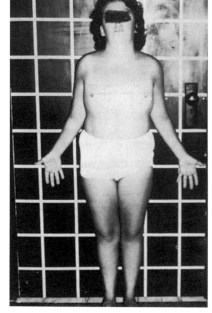

From Sadler TW: The urogenital system. In Lang-mans' Medical Embryology. Baltimore, Williams & Wilkins, 1990, pp 260–296; with permission.

Primary amenorrhea secondary to Turner syndrome

The photo shows a classic patient with Turner syndrome. She has slight webbing of the neck, short stature (notice the doorknob), a broad chest with widely spaced nipples, and lack of breast development. She also has an increased carrying angle at the elbow (**cubitus valgus**).

Pathophysiology

Turner syndrome is usually due to an **absent X chromosome (45 XO)**; rarely, it results from a mosaic pattern or an isochromosome. The syndrome occurs in roughly **1 in 3000 female births.** The ovaries are not formed or functional (this syndrome is sometimes called **gonadal dysgenesis**) and classically are described as "streak" ovaries. Genital development is essentially stagnant after birth, once maternal estrogen is withdrawn, as patients do not make significant amounts of estrogen. Multiple congenital anomalies are associated with Turner syndrome—most classic are **coarctation of the aorta, cystic hygromas** (this patient's "neck tumor"), and **renal anomalies.**

Diagnosis & Treatment

Turner syndrome is most commonly identified when an adolescent **fails to develop secondary sexual characteristics.** It is the **most common cause of primary amenorrhea.** The patient has one or more of the following findings: **short stature,** primary amenorrhea (both invariably present), **lymphedema** of the hands and feet, **webbing of the neck, low posterior hairline, broad chest with widely spaced nipples,** infertility, and **infantile sexual development (breasts, internal and external genitalia, body hair).** *Intellectual function is usually normal,* though patients often have a slightly low nonverbal IQ on standardized testing.

The diagnosis should be confirmed with **chromosomal analysis,** to determine the exact genetic type. This could have important implications for the parents in terms of **genetic counseling.** Rarely, a patient has a Y chromosome; these patients need prophylactic gonadal removal secondary to a markedly **increased risk of gonadal malignancy.**

Treatment is **estrogen replacement therapy** at the time of puberty (generally continued for life) to allow normal secondary sexual characteristics to develop. Patients remain infertile. Many advocate growth hormone to combat short stature, but better proof is still needed.

More High-Yield Facts

Cystic hygroma or coarctation of the aorta are classic for Turner syndrome.

If a Turner syndrome patient is given progesterone, she does *not* experience withdrawal bleeding, due to a lack of estrogen.

Case 10

Gynecology

History

A 34-year-old woman is troubled by profuse, foul-smelling vaginal discharge. The discharge began 4 days ago, but is not associated with fever, dysuria, or vaginal discomfort. The patient is single and has not been sexually active in the last 3 months. She has a history of multiple sexual partners and admits that she does not frequently use condoms. The patient is otherwise healthy and takes no regular medications.

Exam

T: 98.5°F   BP: 122/78   RR: 16/min.   P: 66/min.

The patient is healthy appearing and in no acute distress. Chest and abdominal exams are unremarkable. Pelvic exam reveals no masses. Speculum exam shows a fairly profuse, foul-smelling vaginal discharge that is gray, thin, and watery. There is no erythema, edema, or petechiae formation noted on examination of the vaginal mucosa and cervix. The pH of the discharge is 5.2. When viewed microscopically, unusual-appearing granular epithelial cells are evident (see figure), but few white blood cells. While making a potassium hydroxide preparation of the discharge, you note a peculiar fishy odor; however, no hyphae are identified.

Tests

Hemoglobin: 15 g/dL (normal 12–16)
White blood cell count: 6200/μL (normal 4500–11,000)
Urinalysis: negative for glucose, protein, and bacteria; normal specific gravity

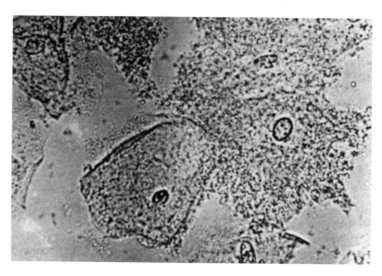

From Brown Jr D, Kaufman RH. In Glass RH (ed): Office Gynecology, 4th ed. Baltimore, Williams & Wilkins, 1993, pp 25–54; with permission.

Bacterial vaginosis (*Gardnerella* vaginitis)

The slide reveals classic **"clue cells,"** which are **epithelial cells with a granular appearance** due to numerous adherent bacteria (gram-negative *Gardnerella* bacilli).

Pathophysiology

Bacterial vaginosis is due to a **disturbance** in the normal vaginal flora. It is not generally considered to be a transmissible infection, though recurrent cases are often linked to the frequency of sexual intercourse. The cause of the flora disturbance is unknown, but the result is overgrowth of *Gardnerella* with resultant symptoms and signs. Bacterial vaginosis has now been linked to **postpartum endometritis,** pelvic infections (pelvic inflammatory disease and posthysterectomy infections), and **preterm labor**.

Diagnosis & Treatment

The classic symptom is a **profuse, watery, foul-smelling, "dirty-gray" discharge**. Dysuria, vaginal burning and itching, and dyspareunia are characteristically *absent*. Patients are not necessarily sexually active and/or promiscuous.

The discharge has a **pH around 5,** contains clue cells and **few to no white blood cells,** and gives a **positive "whiff test,"** which means that when potassium hydroxide is added to the discharge, a fishy odor can be detected.

Treatment is generally with **metronidazole (clindamycin** is an alternative regimen) for approximately 7 days. Either can be given orally or as a vaginal gel.

More High-Yield Facts

Treatment of sexual partners is *not* indicated.

Pregnant women with bacterial vaginosis should be treated. Metronidazole should *not* be used during the **first trimester,** due to concerns over teratogenicity. Screening asymptomatic pregnant women is currently controversial.

Case 11

Gynecology

History

A 33-year-old, nulliparous business executive complains of chronic pelvic pain and the recent development of pain during sexual intercourse. The woman says her pelvic pain began several years ago but has become progressively worse over the years. The pain generally only occurs during menstruation. The patient also mentions increasingly common pre- and postmenstrual spotting. The dyspareunia began several months ago, but has gotten worse. In addition, the patient develops pain during defecation, as she is passing stool. The pain quickly goes away after she finishes her bowel movement, and she denies any change in the color or caliber of her stool. She says she has never mentioned her symptoms before because she is "too busy" at work to be concerned with minor pains.

The woman is sexually active only with her husband. They do not use birth control, as they have been trying to get pregnant for the last 3.5 years. The patient takes no medications and has no other health problems. She had a normal Pap smear 6 months ago.

Exam

T: 98.8°F   BP: 126/80   RR: 12/min.   P: 70/min.

The patient is healthy appearing and in no acute distress. Chest and abdominal exams are unremarkable. Speculum exam is normal, with no discharge identified. Pelvic exam reveals a fixed, retroverted uterus. There is nodularity of the uterosacral ligaments bilaterally, and they are somewhat tender. Both ovaries are somewhat tender and mildly enlarged. No cervical motion tenderness is evident.

Tests

Hemoglobin: 13 g/dL (normal 12–16)
White blood cell count: 6200/μL (normal 4500–11,000)
Thyroid-stimulating hormone level: 2.1 μU/mL (normal 0.5–5.0)
Erythrocyte sedimentation rate (ESR): 8 mm/hr (normal 1–20)
AST: 12 u/L (normal 7–27)
Glucose: 80 mg/dL (normal fasting 70–110 mg/dL)
Urine pregnancy test: negative
Urinalysis: negative for glucose, protein, and bacteria; normal specific gravity

Pathophysiology

Endometriosis is an idiopathic condition in which endometrial glands and stroma are found **outside the uterus,** most commonly in the **ovary,** fallopian tubes, **uterine ligaments,** and/or pelvic peritoneum. Roughly 5–15% of women are affected by this condition to some extent. Endometriosis "implants" can cause multiple symptoms, partly based on their location.

Diagnosis & Treatment

Most women present between the ages of **20 and 35**. Classic symptoms occur in a **nulliparous,** "type A" personality and include **dysmenorrhea, intermenstrual spotting, dyspareunia** (painful intercourse), and **dyschezia** (painful defecation). **Infertility** is another classic presentation, though the mechanism is often unclear. Because the endometrial implants are hormone sensitive, pelvic **symptoms may get worse with menstruation,** as the implants can go through the same cyclical changes as normal endometrial tissue. However, chronic symptoms eventually occur, due to **scarring** and **adhesion** formation (which can affect fertility).

Physical exam may reveal one or more classic findings, including a **fixed, retroverted uterus; nodularity in the uterosacral and other pelvic ligaments;** and **fixed ovaries** (which may cause an adnexal mass). These areas may or may not be tender. In many women, there are no physical findings. A routine infertility work-up, if done, will generally be *negative* in the woman and her partner.

Confirmation of the diagnosis can only be done via **visualization of the implants** with **laparoscopy,** though ultrasound or MRI may suggest the diagnosis. Treatment is variable, depending on symptoms and desire for fertility. **Surgical removal/destruction** of endometrial implants and lysis of adhesions restores fertility in at least 50% of women who are infertile. Medical therapy includes NSAIDs for mild symptoms; **oral contraceptive pills, danazol,** and **GnRH-agonists** (to induce "medical menopause") are other options for more severe symptoms. **Hysterectomy and bilateral salpingo-oophorectomy** is an option for women who do not wish future fertility. Symptoms generally resolve after menopause.

More High-Yield Facts

Endometriosis does *not* cause fever, leukocytosis, or an elevated ESR, distinguishing it from **pelvic inflammatory disease**.

Endometrial implants seen at laparoscopy may resemble "**powder burns**" (brown, flat discolorations) or "**mulberry spots**" (raised, blue-colored).

Case 12

Gynecology

History

A G_5P_5, 46-year-old woman presents with a chief complaint of increasing inter-menstrual spotting and postcoital vaginal bleeding. She also mentions a clear vaginal discharge and wonders if she may have chlamydia, which she had in the past. The patient is currently sexually active with "a few" different partners and has been divorced twice. Her first marriage was at age 16, when she became pregnant. The patient has smoked two packs of cigarettes per day for the last 25 years and drinks alcohol during social occasions. She has no other medical problems, takes no regular medications, and has not been to see a doctor in 10 years.

Exam

T: 98.9°F   BP: 136/86   RR: 14/min.   P: 78/min.

The patient's sclerae are somewhat pale. Chest and abdominal exams are unremarkable. No adnexal or uterine masses are discovered on pelvic exam. Her cervix is somewhat hard and irregular. Speculum exam reveals a friable, ulcerated cervix that bleeds when touched. A punch biopsy is performed (see figure).

Tests

Hemoglobin: 10 g/dL (normal 12–16)
Mean corpuscular volume: 82 μL/cell (normal 80–100)
White blood cell count: 6200/μL (normal 4500–11,000)
Thyroid-stimulating hormone level: 2.1 μU/mL (normal 0.5–5.0)
Urine pregnancy test: negative
Urinalysis: negative for glucose, protein, and bacteria; normal specific gravity

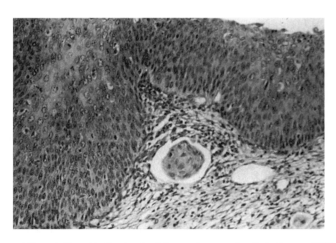

From Jones HW, et al: Novak's Textbook of Gynecology, 11th ed. Baltimore, Williams & Wilkins, 1988, p 684; with permission.

Cervical cancer

The figure shows diffusely atypical, dysplastic epithelial cells, some of which can be seen in a vascular space, indicating invasive cancer.

Pathophysiology

Most cases of cervical cancer are of the **squamous** type and occur at the **squamo-columnar junction** ("transformation zone"). Risk factors for cervical cancer include: **young age (< 20 years old) at first coitus/marriage/pregnancy, multiple sexual partners**/having sex with promiscuous people, **HIV** or **human papillomavirus** (HPV) infection, **smoking, high parity,** divorce, and low socioeconomic status. **Annual Pap smears from the time of first sexual activity** (starting **no later than age 20**) have helped reduce the number of cases of invasive cancer and death.

Diagnosis & Treatment

The mean age at presentation for invasive cancer is **47 years old,** though changes are often detected in the preinvasive stage in younger women who receive regular Pap smears. In the preinvasive stages, patients are **asymptomatic.** Invasive cancer classically causes **abnormal bleeding (postcoital, heavy menstrual bleeding, and/or intermenstrual bleeding)** and a **vaginal discharge** (which may be clear, purulent, and/or malodorous). **Anemia** may also be present. **Weight loss** is a late and ominous finding.

On exam, the cervix may feel **hard or irregular.** The classic description of the cervix is **ulcerated and friable,** often **bleeding with palpation.** Palpable spread may occur into the vagina, uterus, uterine ligaments, or pelvic sidewalls. Early invasive disease (**confined to the cervix**) is generally treated with **hysterectomy,** while **radiation** is generally used for more **advanced disease.** Preinvasive disease can be treated with **conization, cryosurgery, laser, cautery, or LEEP** (excision with a special cautery tool); hysterectomy is also an option.

More High-Yield Facts

Managing an abnormal Pap smear is a common problem. If inflammatory changes or minimal atypia are present, treat any underlying infection and repeat the smear **in 3–6 months** if immediate colposcopy is not performed. For any higher-grade intraepithelial neoplasia or atypia, perform **colposcopy with directed biopsies and endocervical curettage. Diagnostic conization** is needed if the transformation zone cannot be visualized. Further treatment is then based on these results as discussed above.

Only certain HPV serotypes are implicated in cervical cancer, but the list continues to grow longer. **Types 16, 18, 31, 33,** and others (**all higher than 16**) are **carcinogenic,** while **types 6 and 11** cause **genital warts.**

Case 13

Gynecology

History

A 24-year-old woman is suffering painful genital lesions and has been "feeling lousy" for the past 4 days. She describes the pain primarily as intense burning and denies any significant vaginal discharge. The patient says she initially saw a few blisters on her vagina, but they broke open yesterday. She is sexually active with multiple male partners and doesn't always use condoms.

Exam

T: 99.6°F   BP: 118/74   RR: 12/min.   P: 78/min.

The patient is athletic appearing and in no acute distress. Head, neck, chest, and abdominal exams are unremarkable. Examination of the genitals reveals lesions (see figure), which are tender to the touch.

Tests

Hemoglobin: 14 g/dL (normal 12–16)
White blood cell count: 7800/μL (normal 4500–11,000)
Urine pregnancy test: negative
Urinalysis: negative for glucose, protein, and bacteria; normal specific gravity

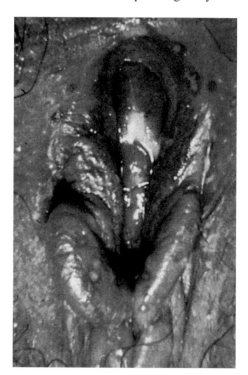

From Jones HW, et al: Novak's Textbook of Gynecology, 11th ed. Baltimore, Williams & Wilkins, 1988, p 585; with permission.

Herpes genitalis

The figure shows the typical gross appearance of multiple shallow ulcers seen with herpes.

Pathophysiology

Herpes genitalis is caused by **herpes simplex virus type II,** a DNA virus that is **sexually transmitted**. Type I causes 10% of cases. Symptoms usually occur within 1 week of exposure, though many patients remain **asymptomatic**. Infection is considered **permanent,** with roughly one-third of affected persons having **recurrent outbreaks** of genital lesions.

Diagnosis & Treatment

Prodromal symptoms, such as **paresthesias** and **burning** in the perineal area, may occur before lesions become visible. Lesions are **painful** and **tender**. **Malaise, low-grade fever,** and **inguinal lymphadenopathy** are fairly common.

The lesions are **multiple** and start out as **vesicles,** which rupture 1–7 days later and leave **shallow ulcers with surrounding erythema**. Small ulcers usually heal **within 2 weeks** without scar formation, though coalescence of smaller lesions may result in a larger lesion that can become infected and/or take several weeks to heal.

Diagnosis can usually be made by the **appearance** of the lesions, but a cytologic ("**Tzanck**") smear often reveals the classic appearance of **multinucleated cells with intranuclear (Cowdry) inclusion bodies**. **Culture** of vesicle fluid or material taken from the base of an ulcer is considered the **gold standard** when diagnostic confirmation is needed.

Treatment includes analgesics and **acyclovir, valacyclovir, or famciclovir** for 7–10 days. Those with recurrences can be maintained on a lower **daily suppressive dose**. Advise use of **condoms** at all times, as transmission may occur **even in the asymptomatic phase,** and sex should be **avoided completely** when active lesions are present.

More High-Yield Facts

Management of pregnant women with herpes genitalis: women should be examined **at the time of labor**. If lesions are present, a **cesarean section** is generally recommended to prevent maternal-fetal transmission. If no lesions are present at the time of labor, **vaginal delivery** is generally preferred.

Herpes infection may play a role in the development of **cervical cancer**.

Gynecology

History

A 16-year-old girl presents with a chief complaint of missing her period. She states that her last period was 3 months ago, and her periods were somewhat irregular in the few months before that. From the ages of 13 to 15, however, the patient's menstrual cycles were quite regular.

The patient also mentions feeling bloated and asks about medications to prevent water retention. She does modeling for a local fashion designer when not in school, where she is a straight "A" student. She has not been sexually active for the last year, mentioning that she needs to lose a few pounds before she'll be able to find a boyfriend. She has no other medical conditions and takes no medications.

Exam

T: 96.6°F   BP: 108/66   RR: 12/min.   P: 54/min.

The patient is wearing baggy clothes, but when she removes her sweater for the chest examination, you note that she is markedly emaciated. Review of the nurse's notes indicates that her weight is well below the 5th percentile for her height, though her height is normal. Her sclerae are slightly pale. Cardiac exam is remarkable only for bradycardia. Pelvic exam reveals a normal uterus and ovaries. Speculum exam is unremarkable. Secondary sexual characteristics are appropriate for age.

Tests

Hemoglobin: 10 g/dL (normal 12–16)
White blood cell count: 3800/μL (normal 4500–11,000)
Urine pregnancy test: negative
HIV test: negative
Luteinizing hormone (LH) level: 2.3 mU/mL (normal 2.5–40)
Follicle-stimulating hormone (FSH) level: 4.5 mU/mL (normal 5–40)
Estradiol: 20 pg/mL (normal 30–360)
Urinalysis: negative for glucose, protein, and bacteria; normal specific gravity

Pathophysiology

Anorexia nervosa is a psychiatric disorder that can cause severe physiologic disturbances due to **chronic malnutrition**. As with most psychiatric disorders, the cause is poorly understood, but anorexia is very common in the U.S., occurring in roughly **1% of female teenagers**. However, it is extremely rare in areas with food shortage, implicating **social factors**. Females comprise **95% of patients.** **Half** of affected patients also have **bulimia**.

Diagnosis & Treatment

Affected persons are generally **teenage females** who are **intelligent** and **meticulous,** with high standards for achievement. Classic patient activities include **ballet** and **modeling** (where body habitus is stressed). Those affected do not mention their disorder and usually only present for other symptoms (**amenorrhea, bloating,** constipation) or illnesses, or are **forced** to seek medical attention by their parents.

The DSM-IV criteria for diagnosis include a **distorted sense of body image** (patients think they are fat even though emaciated), **failure to maintain at least 85% of ideal body weight, intense fear of gaining weight,** and **amenorrhea for at least three menstrual cycles**. Laboratory findings include **low LH, FSH, and estrogens** (hypothalamic depression from starvation is thought to be partly responsible for the amenorrhea), **anemia, leukopenia,** and depressed thyroxine levels. **Bradycardia** and **hypothermia** may also occur. Severe **electrolyte disturbances** and **cardiac arrhythmias** are most commonly seen in the presence of coexisting bulimia.

Treatment is difficult, as patients are **manipulative** and do not want to gain weight. **Hospitalization** to treat severe malnutrition, with hyperalimentation in some cases, is only a short-term solution. **Long-term psychotherapy** and antidepressants for any coexisting depression are necessary to help change the patient's attitudes toward food and weight, and improve her distorted sense of body image. **Death may occur in extreme cases** from complications of **malnutrition**.

More High-Yield Facts

Watch for **enamel erosion in the back of the teeth** and **erosion of the skin over the knuckles** in cases of coexisting (or isolated) **bulimia**. These findings are due to patients repeatedly inducing vomiting by sticking their fingers down their throat. Bulimia is characterized by episodes of "**binging**" (uncontrollable eating) alternating with episodes of "**purging**" (self-induced vomiting, laxative or diuretic abuse, rigorous exercise, or fasting). These patients also have a **disturbed sense of body image**.

Gynecology

History

A 16-year-old girl is experiencing abdominal pain and nausea, and she feels as though she has a fever. She says the pain came on gradually over the past few days, but became worse in the last 24 hours, as the nausea and fever developed. She also mentions a scanty, yellowish vaginal discharge, which was much worse a few weeks ago, but has gotten better on its own. The patient is sexually active, had three different male partners over the past year, and rarely uses condoms. She does not think she is pregnant because she began menstruating 3 days ago.

Exam

T: 102.1°F   BP: 116/78   RR: 16/min.   P: 94/min.

The patient is slightly diaphoretic and uncomfortable appearing. Her sclerae appear normal, and lymphadenopathy is absent. Chest and upper abdominal exams are unremarkable. The patient has severe tenderness to palpation in both lower quadrants, without peritoneal signs. Bowel sounds are slightly decreased, but present. Pelvic exam reveals cervical tenderness when the cervix is manually manipulated and bilateral adnexal tenderness. Speculum examination reveals a purulent cervical discharge.

Tests

Hemoglobin: 13 g/dL (normal 12–16)
White blood cell count: 17,800/µL (normal 4500–11,000)
Neutrophils: 85%
Urine pregnancy test: negative
Erythrocyte sedimentation rate (ESR): 74 mm/hr (normal 1–20)
Urinalysis: negative for glucose, protein, and bacteria; normal specific gravity

Pelvic inflammatory disease (PID)

Pathophysiology

Pelvic inflammatory disease is a term used to describe infection of the upper genital tract, including the uterine cavity (**endometritis**), parauterine tissues/ligaments (**parametritis**), fallopian tubes (**salpingitis**), ovaries (involved in **tubo-ovarian abscesses**), and pelvic peritoneum (**peritonitis**). Most cases are due to ascending sexually transmitted infections, classically *Neisseria gonorrhoeae* and *Chlamydia trachomatis,* though a **polymicrobial** infection is usually present. Sequelae of PID include sepsis, **infertility,** chronic pelvic pain, dyspareunia, pelvic adhesions, and **ectopic pregnancy**.

Diagnosis & Treatment

Patients usually present between **15 and 30 years old,** the ages when sexually transmitted diseases are most prevalent, and are **sexually active (often with multiple partners)**. Classic symptoms include **lower abdominal or pelvic pain, vaginal discharge, nausea,** and **dysuria**.

The textbook diagnosis of PID requires **abdominal tenderness, cervical motion tenderness, and adnexal tenderness**. In addition, one or more of the following should be present: **elevated ESR/C-reactive protein, leukocytosis** (usually with an increased neutrophil count/"left shift"), **purulent cervical discharge,** and **fever**. A **fluctuant adnexal mass** often indicates the presence of a tubo-ovarian abscess.

Treatment is inpatient intravenous **antibiotics** (outpatient treatment okay for mild symptoms in a reliable patient, but be conservative on the boards). Antibiotics must cover chlamydia, gonorrhea, **gram-negative rods** (e.g., *E. coli*), and **anaerobes** (e.g., *Bacteroides*). A popular current regimen is cefotetan or cefoxitin **plus** doxycycline. Treat sexual partners. Patients with a tubo-ovarian abscess need surgery if they do not respond to antibiotics within 72 hours, but **initial medical management is preferred** (different from other types of abscesses that often require drainage first).

More High-Yield Facts

Patients with an **intrauterine device (IUD)** have a higher risk of PID, but the causative organism is classically *Actinomyces israelii*. This risk + the increased risk of ectopic pregnancy with IUDs = *don't prescribe an IUD for contraception in women under age 35, promiscuous women, or those desiring future fertility.*

Case 16

Gynecology

History

A G_3P_3, 41-year-old woman is troubled by increasingly heavy, difficult, and painful menstrual periods. The patient states that over the last several months, her volume of menstrual flow has increased steadily, though her cycles continue to be regular. She also complains of increasing colicky pain during menstruation that has become almost intolerable. The patient denies vaginal discharge or fever, and is only sexually active with her husband of 25 years. She has no other medical conditions, and her only regular medication is ibuprofen during menstruation, which no longer relieves her symptoms effectively. The patient does not smoke or use drugs, and drinks alcohol only on rare social occasions.

The patient mentions that she went to see another doctor 2 months ago and had a Pap smear and dilation and curettage performed, which were both negative. She was told to take ibuprofen and reduce her stress level. She is coming to you for a second opinion.

Exam

T: 98.1°F   BP: 128/84   RR: 14/min.   P: 76/min.

The patient is healthy appearing and in no acute distress. Her sclerae are some-what pale. Chest and abdominal examinations are unremarkable. Pelvic exam reveals a symmetrically enlarged, smooth uterus with a boggy consistency that is somewhat tender during palpation. No adnexal masses are appreciated. Speculum exam is unremarkable.

Tests

Hemoglobin: 11 g/dL (normal 12–16)
Mean corpuscular volume: 80 μm/cell (normal 80–100)
Ferritin level: 20 μg/L (normal 20–200)
White blood cell count: 8000/μL (normal 4500–11,000)
Urine pregnancy test: negative
Erythrocyte sedimentation rate: 14 mm/hr (normal 1–20)
Urinalysis: negative for glucose, protein, and bacteria; normal specific gravity

Pathophysiology

Adenomyosis is defined as the presence of endometrial glands and stroma within the uterine musculature. The condition is a "cousin" to endometriosis, in which endometrial glands are present outside the uterus (15% of patients with adenomyosis also have endometriosis). The exact etiology is unknown. Patients with this condition may or may not have symptoms. It is thought that roughly 15% of women develop some degree of adenomyosis in their late 30s and early 40s.

Diagnosis & Treatment

Patients usually present between **35 and 45 years old,** which is older than the typical age of presentation with endometriosis. Classic symptoms include **dysmenorrhea** (painful menstruation, often described as **colicky** or **crampy pain**) and **menorrhagia** (increased amount of menstrual flow). Adenomyosis is also a fairly common cause of **chronic pelvic pain** in the older, reproductive-age female.

The classic physical finding is a **symmetrically enlarged, smooth uterus with a boggy** ("squishy") **consistency** that may be **tender to palpation,** helping to distinguish this condition from a fibroid uterus. Many cases are not discovered until a hysterectomy is performed for chronic pelvic pain. **Ultrasound** can occasionally make the diagnosis. **MRI** has recently shown promise and fairly high sensitivity in making the diagnosis, though it is *not* a cost-effective screening tool at this time.

Treatment is fairly limited and includes **analgesics** initially. If analgesics fail, **hysterectomy** is often advised. If women can hold out until menopause, symptoms generally **regress** spontaneously. **GnRH-agonists** may help, but are expensive and have multiple side effects.

More High-Yield Facts

Women who present with symptoms of adenomyosis (menorrhagia, dysmenorrhea) need a **dilatation and curettage (D&C)** to exclude **endometrial carcinoma.**

There is some evidence to suggest that **prior pregnancy** and a **history of uterine surgery** (including c-sections, D&C, and tubal ligation) are risk factors for adenomyosis.

Case 17

Gynecology

History

A 19-year-old woman is suffering from "a bad case of the flu." Her symptoms include nausea, vomiting, fever, shaking chills, muscle pain, headache, profuse and watery diarrhea, and skin rash. The patient states that her symptoms developed rapidly yesterday evening and continue to get worse. She finished her menstrual period yesterday, which was not unusual in any way, except that she had used tampons for the first time.

The patient is otherwise usually in excellent health, has no recent sick contacts, takes no regular medications, and does not smoke, drink alcohol, or use drugs. She is not currently sexually active.

Exam

T: 104.1°F   BP: 104/56   RR: 22/min.   P: 116/min.

The patient is toxic appearing and diaphoretic. Her skin is diffusely and intensely erythematous and hot. The sclerae are anicteric. Chest and abdominal exams are unremarkable. Pelvic exam reveals a macerated tampon within the vagina, which surprises the patient, as she did not know it was there. No adnexal or uterine masses are appreciated. The vaginal mucosa has an inflamed beefy-red appearance. When the patient stands up at the end of the exam, she mentions that she feels quite light-headed and grabs onto the edge of the examination table to keep from falling down.

Tests

Hemoglobin: 14 g/dL (normal 12–16)
White blood cell (WBC) count: 12,900/µL (normal 4500–11,000)
Platelet count: 50,000/µL (normal 150,000–400,000)
Urine pregnancy test: negative
Blood urea nitrogen (BUN): 34 mg/dL (normal 8–25)
Creatinine: 1.8 mg/dL (normal 0.6–1.5)
Creatine phosphokinase (CPK): 536 u/L (normal 17–148)
CK-MB fraction: 3% (normal < 5%)
Urinalysis: negative for glucose, protein, and bacteria; moderate (2+) WBCs;
    elevated specific gravity

Pathophysiology

TSS is due to the production and absorption of a **bacterial exotoxin** (TSS toxin) usually produced by certain strains of *Staphylococcus aureus* (sometimes by *Streptococcus pyogenes*). The classic cause is colonization of a vaginal tampon that is left in too long, though colonization of other intravaginal objects (e.g., contraceptive sponge), **wounds** (including surgical wounds), and essentially any *S. aureus* infection can also result in this condition.

The systemic absorption of the toxin (a superantigen) causes exuberant **cytokine release,** which causes most of the signs and symptoms of TSS.

Diagnosis & Treatment

The epidemiology of TSS is changing, but the classic patient is still a **younger woman using tampons**. In this setting, symptoms generally start at the end of menstruation. Classic symptoms are often nonspecific and include **nausea, vomiting, fever, shaking chills, myalgia, headache, profuse** and **watery diarrhea,** and a **skin rash** ("sunburn rash").

Classic physical findings include **high fever (> 102° F), diffuse and intense skin erythema, hypotension, altered mental status,** and **hyperemia** of the **conjunctiva, oropharynx,** and/or **vagina.** Lab findings include elevated **CPK, leukocytosis, azotemia** (elevated BUN/creatinine), elevated **liver function tests, thrombocytopenia,** and **sterile pyuria** (WBCs in the urine without evidence of a urinary tract infection). **Desquamation of the skin,** classically affecting the **palms** and **soles** of the feet, is the physical finding that gives the case away. Unfortunately, this doesn't occur until 1 to 2 weeks after the onset of the illness (usually during recovery).

Initial treatment involves **removing** and **culturing the source of contamination** (tampon or other foreign body); also drain and debride any purulent areas. Supportive care such as **IV fluids** and shock management is given at the same time as **anti-staphylococcal antibiotics** (pull out the "big-gun" antibiotics for this life-threatening infection).

More High-Yield Facts

Staphylococcal "scalded skin" syndrome is similar to TSS and is also caused by a toxin-secreting strain of *S. aureus,* but classically occurs in **infants** and immunosuppressed patients after an impetigo-type rash. It also tends to cause more widespread skin desquamation earlier in the course of the illness. Treatment is similar, and mortality is rare.

Case 18

Gynecology

History

A 22-year-old woman presents with a chief complaint of painless lesions on her vagina. She says the lesions began to appear roughly 1 week ago, and have grown rather quickly. The patient denies pain, itching, burning, vaginal discharge, and dysuria. She is sexually active and has had two male sexual partners in the past year. She says her use of condoms is "occasional." She is otherwise in good health and denies any history of sexually transmitted diseases. Her only regular medication is oral contraceptive pills.

Exam

T: 98.4°F   BP: 120/82   RR: 14/min.   P: 66/min.

The patient appears healthy and is in no acute distress. Her physical exam is mostly unremarkable. Pelvic exam reveals normal uterus and adnexa bilaterally, but examination of the perineum reveals multiple soft, nontender lesions (see figure). Speculum exam is normal, and no cervical lesions are identified.

Tests

Hemoglobin: 14 g/dL (normal 12–16)

White blood cell count: 5900/μL (normal 4500–11,000)

Urine pregnancy test: negative

Glucose level: 96 mg/dL (normal fasting: 70–110)

VDRL serologic syphilis test: negative

Urinalysis: negative for glucose, protein, and bacteria; normal specific gravity

Pap smear: mild koilocytic atypia

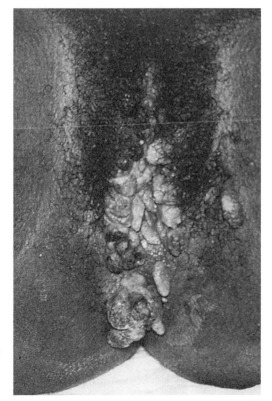

From Brown Jr D, Kaufman RH. In Glass RH (ed): Office Gynecology, 4th ed. Baltimore, Williams & Wilkins, 1993, pp 25–54; with permission.

Condyloma acuminata

Condyloma acuminata is associated with **genital** or **venereal warts**. The figure shows the classic appearance of the lesions.

Pathophysiology

Condyloma acuminata are due to infection with certain serotypes of the sexually transmitted human papillomavirus (HPV), a **papovavirus**. HPV **serotypes 6 and 11** are classically associated with genital warts, while **serotypes 16,18, 31, 33,** and others are associated with the development of **cervical cancer**. Different serotypes of HPV are responsible for non-sexually transmitted warts on other parts of the body.

Diagnosis & Treatment

As with most sexually transmitted diseases, the classic patient is between **15 and 30 years old** at the time of presentation. The lesions are usually multiple and can occur on the **vulva, perineum, vagina, cervix,** and/or **anus,** partly depending on sexual practices. They are **painless** and often **cause no symptoms** other than their undesirable appearance. A Pap smear that reveals **koilocytic atypia** generally indicates infection with HPV.

The lesions are **soft, moist, nontender,** and often **pinkish** or reddish in color. They generally appear in **clusters** and may range from small, nodular swellings to the classic **large, pedunculated, "cauliflower-like"** lesions. In women who are pregnant, diabetic, immunosuppressed, or taking oral contraceptive pills, the lesions often grow *rapidly* and to a larger size.

There are multiple treatments available for the lesions. A **Pap smear should be obtained in all women first,** as neoplastic cervical changes from HPV may change the management (as may pregnancy). Patients can be given **podophyllin, podofilox, or imiquimod** for topical application. In addition, physician application of concentrated **podophyllin** or **trichloroacetic acid,** intralesional **interferon** injection, **cryotherapy,** electrocautery, laser therapy, and surgery are options. Recurrence is common, and **sexual partners** should be **screened and treated**. Lesions may become malignant (rarely); excisional biopsy is needed if suspicious.

More High-Yield Facts

Condyloma acuminata must be differentiated from **condyloma lata,** which are anogenital warts that occur in **secondary syphilis**. Condyloma lata are usually more **flat-topped** and **papular** in appearance. In some cases, **biopsy** may be needed to distinguish the two (condyloma lata contain large numbers of **spirochetes** that can be visualized with dark-field microscopy).

Though the serotypes that cause warts are different, women are often **coinfected** with carcinogenic serotypes and need close follow-up with at least **annual Pap smears** to detect cytologic atypia or early cervical cancer.

Case 19
Gynecology

History

A 62-year-old woman is seeking medical advice for abnormal vaginal bleeding and fatigue. She says that the bleeding, with occasional passing of blood clots, has been occurring intermittently for 7–8 weeks. She went through menopause at age 59 and does not take hormone replacement therapy. The patient mentions that she always had irregular, infrequent periods when she used to menstruate. She has no children.

The woman's past medical history is significant for obesity, type II diabetes, hypertension, and gallstones that required cholecystectomy 8 years ago. She takes glipizide and metoprolol. She proudly mentions that she recently lost some weight, but upon questioning, the patient admits that she hasn't changed her diet or level of physical activity. She has a strong family history of breast cancer, but denies any breast lumps or discharge.

Exam

T: 99.2°F   BP: 150/92   RR: 18/min.   P: 76/min.

The woman is obese but in no acute distress. Head, neck, breast, chest, and abdominal exams are unremarkable, except for mild scleral pallor. Pelvic exam reveals a slightly enlarged, irregular uterus with unusual firmness in the region of the internal cervical os. The external genitalia are normal. Speculum exam shows an abnormally patent cervical os with a small, fresh blood clot protruding from it. No cervical erosion or friability is noted.

Tests

Hemoglobin: 10 g/dL (normal 12–16)
Mean corpuscular volume: 82 μm/cell (normal 80–100)
White blood cell count: 6700/μL (normal 4500–11,000)
Platelet count: 450,000/μL (normal 150,000–400,000)
Urine pregnancy test: negative
Glucose level: 166 mg/dL (normal fasting: 70–110)
Urinalysis: negative for glucose, protein, and bacteria; normal specific gravity

Pathophysiology

Endometrial cancer is the **most common gynecologic cancer** and **the fourth most common cancer in women** overall. Most cases are due to **adenocarcinoma**. Risk factors include **obesity, nulliparity, late menopause, diabetes, hypertension, gallbladder disease,** and chronic **unopposed estrogen stimulation** (e.g., estrogen-replacement therapy without progesterone, anovulatory cycles, estrogen-secreting neoplasms). A history (or family history) of breast, colon, or ovarian cancer also increases the risk of endometrial cancer.

Diagnosis & Treatment

Most women present between the ages of **50 to 65** (60 is the median age). The classic complaint is **abnormal vaginal bleeding,** which can include menorrhagia and intermenstrual spotting in premenopausal women. **Weight loss** may indicate more advanced disease.

Physical exam is often entirely normal, but may reveal **uterine enlargement,** a **pelvic mass, hardening/expansion/irregularity** of the **uterus** or **cervix,** and/or a **patent cervical os**. Blood and/or blood clots may be seen coming from the os in some cases.

In the investigation of abnormal vaginal bleeding of unknown cause, especially in a postmenopausal female, a **Pap smear, endocervical curettage,** and **endometrial biopsy** should be performed. **Hysteroscopy** and **dilation and curettage** may be performed if the biopsy is negative or equivocal. **Ultrasound** is commonly used to examine the endometrium and look for other pelvic abnormalities.

Treatment is generally **surgical** (hysterectomy with bilateral salpingo-oophorectomy and lymph node dissection), with **adjuvant radiation therapy** when the cancer has invaded beyond the superficial myometrium. More advanced disease (spread outside uterus) is generally treated with **medical therapy** (hormonal therapy and chemotherapy), with surgery mainly **palliative** in this setting.

More High-Yield Facts

Vaginal bleeding in a postmenopausal woman without an obvious cause is endometrial cancer *"until proven otherwise."*

Progesterone + estrogen for postmenopausal hormone replacement therapy = no increased risk of endometrial cancer. A woman *doesn't* need progesterone with her estrogen therapy if she has *no uterus,* but a woman with a uterus should generally receive progesterone *and* estrogen.

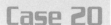

Case 20

Gynecology

History

A 34-year-old woman presents with vaginal itching, irritation, and discomfort, along with a thick, whitish discharge. She says the symptoms started roughly 1 week ago. The patient mentions taking amoxicillin 2 weeks ago for a urinary tract infection. She is sexually active only with her husband and denies any history of sexually transmitted diseases. She mentions that sex has become painful in the last few days because of worsening vaginal irritation. Past medical history is significant for obesity and type II diabetes mellitus. Her only regular medications are metformin and oral contraceptive pills.

Exam

T: 98.7°F   BP: 130/86   RR: 16/min.   P: 78/min.

The woman is obese, but in no acute distress. The non-gynecologic portion of the exam is unremarkable. Pelvic exam reveals normal external genitalia, and no palpable abnormalities in the uterus or adnexae. Speculum exam shows an exquisitely tender, erythematous, and edematous-appearing vulva and vagina. The cervix is normal in appearance. A white, thick, curdy vaginal discharge that resembles cottage cheese covers much of the vaginal mucosa. The discharge is not malodorous. A potassium hydroxide slide of the discharge is prepared (see figure).

Tests

Hemoglobin: 14 g/dL (normal 12–16)   WBCs: 6700/μL (normal 4500–11,000)
Platelets: 300,000/μL   Urine pregnancy test: negative
Glucose level: 246 mg/dL (normal fasting 70–110)
Urinalysis: positive for glucose; negative for protein and bacteria

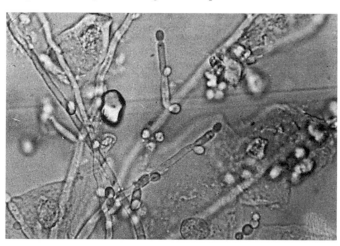

From Brown Jr D, Kaufman RH. In Glass RH (ed): Office Gynecology, 4th ed. Baltimore, Williams & Wilkins, 1993, pp 25–54; with permission.

Vulvovaginitis secondary to candidiasis

The slide reveals the classic appearance of a budding yeast with pseudohyphae ("yeast infection").

Pathophysiology

Candidiasis is caused by the yeast *Candida,* usually **C. albicans**. It typically develops in normal women and generally is not sexually transmitted; rather, it is considered a disturbance in the normal vaginal flora. **Risk factors** for candidiasis include **diabetes, recent antibiotic use, oral contraceptive pills, immunosuppression/ corticosteroid use,** and **pregnancy**. Roughly **75% of all women** will experience at least one vaginal yeast infection during their lifetime.

Diagnosis & Treatment

The classic patient is a **reproductive-age female,** but children and postmenopausal females can also be affected. The risk factors discussed above may or may not be present, as this is a very common condition. The classic symptoms include **vaginal irritation** and **itching;** a thick, white **vaginal discharge;** and, often, **dyspareunia**.

Physical findings include **vulvar and vaginal tenderness, erythema, and edema**. The discharge is **thick, white, and curd-like/cheesy,** with a pH of around **4.5**. It is classically described as resembling **cottage cheese**. Some of the discharge is often **adherent to the vaginal walls**. The discharge is characteristically *not* malodorous. A slide made after treating the discharge with potassium hydroxide ("**KOH prep**") reveals the typical **oval, budding yeast** and branching **pseudohyphae**. Culture is the **gold standard** for diagnosis, but is rarely needed.

Multiple treatments are available. Most popular with patients is a **1-day oral regimen** using **fluconazole** or itraconazole. **Intravaginal topical application** of an antifungal (e.g., **clotrimazole, miconazole,** terconazole, butoconazole, nystatin) is another option.

More High-Yield Facts

In cases of recurrent candidiasis, consider the possibility of underlying **diabetes** or **immunosuppresive disorder** (e.g., AIDS), especially if extravaginal candidiasis (e.g., thrush) also occurs. In some recurrent cases, treatment of sexual partners may result in cure.

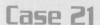

Case 21

Gynecology

History

A 26-year-old woman has been troubled by lower abdominal heaviness and pressure, primarily on the left side, for the past 3 months. She denies any menstrual irregularities and says she just finished her most recent menstrual period 1 week ago. She has had no change in bowel or urinary habits and denies weight loss or other constitutional symptoms. The patient is sexually active only with her fiancée and denies any history or symptoms of sexually transmitted diseases. The patient smokes, drinks alcohol on occasion, and denies using illicit drugs. She has no significant past medical history and takes no regular medications.

Exam

T: 98.9°F   BP: 124/80   RR: 14/min.   P: 70/min.

The woman is healthy appearing and in no acute distress. Head and chest exams are unremarkable. She has some discomfort to deep palpation in the left lower quadrant, but no rebound tenderness or guarding. Bowel sounds are normal. Pelvic exam reveals an 8-centimeter, left adnexal mass. The mass is nontender, well circumscribed, round, and mobile. The uterus and right adnexa are normal. Speculum exam and external genitalia exam are normal, and no vaginal discharge is identified.

Tests

Hemoglobin: 15 g/dL (normal 12–16)
White blood cell count: 6700/μL (normal 4500–11,000)
Platelet count: 300,000/μL (normal 150,000–400,000)
Urine pregnancy test: negative
Urinalysis: negative for glucose, protein, white blood cells, and bacteria
Pelvic ultrasound: heterogeneous, well-circumscribed mass with both cystic and
    solid components; various densities, including fluid, fat, and focal areas of
    well-circumscribed, dense calcification

Benign cystic teratoma

Benign cystic teratoma is also referred to as mature teratoma or dermoid cyst.

Pathophysiology

Dermoid cysts are the **most common ovarian neoplasms** and are **benign**. They are considered **germ cell tumors** (as opposed to epithelial tumors such as cystadenomas/cystadenocarcinomas). The interesting thing about these tumors is that they often contain **well-differentiated** tissues from all three germ cell layers (ectoderm, endoderm, and mesoderm), though ectodermal elements (**skin, hair, teeth**) generally predominate. In 15% of cases, the tumor is **bilateral**. In the malignant form of teratoma, or immature teratoma, the different tissue elements are **poorly differentiated**.

Diagnosis & Treatment

A teratoma generally presents in the same fashion as any benign ovarian mass. Often there are **no symptoms** until the mass becomes large enough to cause **pressure, heaviness,** or **pain** in the pelvis or lower abdomen. The mass may press on the bladder or rectum and cause a **change in bowel or urinary habits** (e.g., urinary frequency). Occasionally, patients present with severe, acute pain due to **tumor rupture** or **ovarian torsion**.

The diagnosis can sometimes be made prior to surgery with pelvic **ultrasound** or **CT scan,** due to the unique collection of tissues contained in the tumor. A cystic, well-circumscribed mass containing **fat, fluid, higher-density soft tissue,** and focal areas of **calcification** (often representing **tooth formation**) can confidently be called a teratoma, as no other tumor has this many different types of tissue within it. An extremely rare presentation (seen only on the boards or talked about on rounds!) is **struma ovarii,** which is hyperthyroidism caused by functioning thyroid tissue within a teratoma.

Because malignant degeneration rarely occurs in these tumors and the histology is not certain prior to surgery, **surgical resection** is the treatment of choice (unilateral salpingo-oopherectomy is generally performed) and is **curative**.

More High-Yield Facts

Other germ cell tumors include **yolk sac tumors (elevated alpha-fetoprotein levels), choriocarcinomas (elevated human chorionic gonadotropin levels),** and **dysgerminomas.** These are quite rare and often malignant.

Gynecology

History

An 18-year-old woman presents with a chief complaint of painless "bumps" on her genitals. She says the bumps developed a week ago. She denies fever, vaginal discharge, dysuria, and pain. The patient is in good health and has no medical problems; she takes no regular medications. She is sexually active and has had multiple partners over the last few months. The patient had chlamydia in the past, which was treated.

Exam

T: 98.8°F   BP: 118/80   RR: 12/min.   P: 64/min.

The woman is healthy appearing and in no acute distress. Head, chest, and abdominal exams are unremarkable. The lesions are evident on external genitalia exam (see figure). Several discrete inguinal nodes are enlarged, fairly firm, and nontender. Pelvic and speculum examinations are normal, with no masses or discharge.

Tests

Hemoglobin: 13 g/dL (normal 12–16)
White blood cell count: 6700/μL (normal 4500–11,000)
AST: 9 u/L (normal 1–27)
Urine pregnancy test: negative
Urinalysis: negative for glucose, protein, white blood cells, and bacteria.
VDRL syphilis test: positive

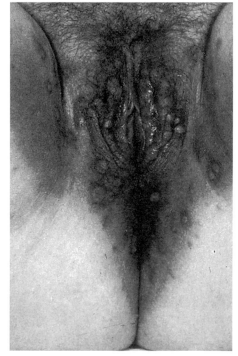

From Eschenbach DA. In Scott JR, et al (eds): Danforth's Obstetrics and Gynecology, 7th ed. Philadelphia, Lippincott, 1988, pp 641–664; with permission.

Syphilis, secondary stage

The photo shows condyloma lata.

Pathophysiology

Syphilis is a sexually transmitted disease caused by the bacteria *Treponema pallidum,* a spirochete. The disease is divided into four stages: primary, secondary, latent, and tertiary. Without treatment, syphilis can disseminate and affect any part of the body. There is **no known way** to culture the organism.

Diagnosis & Treatment

Patients may present at any stage. Most are sexually promiscuous. The *primary* stage occurs roughly **1 month** after exposure and causes a **red papule** that soon erodes to form a **painless ulcer** (chancre). Chancres usually are **single** and have an **indurated base** and a small "collar" of well-circumscribed **surrounding erythema**. Nontender, discrete **inguinal lymphadenopathy** is common. The chancre resolves without treatment in 4 to 8 weeks.

Without treatment, *secondary* syphilis usually occurs soon after the chancre goes away. Findings include **constitutional symptoms, lymphadenopathy,** maculopapular **skin rashes** (classically affecting the **palms**), and **condyloma lata,** which can usually be distinguished from condyloma acuminata by appearance. Latent syphilis is an **asymptomatic phase** that may last for years. *Tertiary* syphilis primarily affects the **central nervous system** (dementia, loss of sensation from posterior column involvement) and the **cardiovascular system** (aortic insufficiency). It is now rather rare.

Diagnosis depends on the stage. Chancres and secondary-stage skin lesions often **contain *T. pallidum* spirochetes,** which can be visualized using **darkfield microscopy**. Serologic tests are either **screening** (VDRL, RPR; these tests are nonspecific, give false positives, and **become negative again after treatment**) or **confirmatory** (FTA-Abs, MHA-TP; **more specific, stay positive for life** after treatment). If you suspect syphilis, order a screening test first, then a confirmatory test if the screening test is positive.

Treatment is a single IM benzathine **penicillin** injection for primary cases (oral penicillin is an alternative), with longer treatment for later stages. The **Jarisch-Herxheimer** reaction (fever, sweating, malaise) may occur in the first day of treatment (don't confuse with an allergic penicillin reaction).

More High-Yield Facts

With a false-positive VDRL/RPR, think of **lupus** or other collagen vascular disorders, such as the **antiphospholipid antibody syndrome**.

Diagnosis of CNS involvement requires a **lumbar puncture** and is more common in those with **HIV,** who also have more rapid progression.

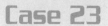

Case 23

Gynecology

History

A 20-year-old woman walks into the emergency department clutching her torn blouse and appearing disoriented. She is brought into an examination room and suddenly begins crying while being questioned about her symptoms. The patient says she was attacked and raped by a man she had just met a few hours before at a party. She believes the attack was her fault and begs you not to tell her mother. Several times during the interview, the patient stares off into space, seeming pre-occupied.

Exam

T: 98.8°F   BP: 122/80   RR: 14/min.   P: 84/min.

The woman is disheveled but calm during most of the examination. She has a bruise on the side of her face, but no lacerations. Chest and abdominal exams are unremarkable. Pelvic exam reveals dried blood and semen on her inner thighs and torn underwear. The patient again begins sobbing loudly and says that she wants to die.

Tests

Hemoglobin: 13 g/dL (normal 12–16)
White blood cell count: 6700/μL (normal 4500–11,000)
AST: 9 u/L (normal 1–27)
Urine pregnancy test: negative
Urinalysis: negative for glucose, protein, white blood cells, and bacteria.

Rape

Rape is the most severe form of sexual assault.

Pathophysiology

Rape occurs when a person (usually a woman) is forced to have sexual intercourse **against her will**. It is estimated that **1 in 6** women will be raped during their lifetime, though **only 50% of rapes are reported**. Women between the ages of **10 and 29** are at highest risk of being raped. In **50%** of cases, the rapist is **known to the victim**. Rape is a crime of violence, and **nonsexual violence** commonly accompanies the rape act. Most rapists are **25- to 44-year-old males,** and they attack women of their own race. **Alcohol** is involved in one-third of cases. Most attacks are **premeditated**.

Diagnosis & Treatment

Women experience both **short and long-term effects** (the **rape trauma syndrome**) from a rape. Initial calm, with inattention and preoccupation, may turn into shock, disbelief, fear, guilt, and shame. Somatic symptoms (headaches, irritable bowel syndrome), behavioral problems, and sexual dysfunction are common long-term sequelae.

When a rape victim presents for acute care, attention must be paid to her **physical *and* psychological needs**. In addition, an accurate history, physical exam, and evidence collection must be carried out for **legal** purposes. **Informed consent** is required for the examination and evidence collection. A detailed search for and documentation of any traumatic injuries is needed.

Standard "**rape kits**" are available to assist with collection of loose hair, debris, cleanings from under the fingernails, clothing, saliva, blood stains, and semen (can be visualized with a **Wood's light**). Baseline labs include syphilis, hepatitis B, and HIV **serology;** a **pregnancy test;** drug/alcohol levels; and oral/cervical/anal **cultures** for sexually transmitted diseases (STDs).

Offer **prophylaxis** for STDs and **postcoital contraception** with high-dose oral contraceptives. **Give tetanus** prophylaxis for lacerations in the absence of a recent booster. HIV prophylaxis may be appropriate, and offer the **hepatitis B** vaccine if prior vaccination is lacking. Professional psychological or **psychiatric consultation** should also be made available in the acute setting. **Group counseling** with other victims is helpful to some. Arrange a follow-up exam to retest for pregnancy and STDs.

More High-Yield Facts

Rape is a well-known cause of **posttraumatic stress disorder**. Patients repeatedly **reexperience the attack** in nightmares or **flashbacks; try to avoid thinking about the attack;** and develop **memory problems, poor concentration, insomnia,** or **depression** as a result.

Case 24

Obstetrics

History

A 17-year-old girl is concerned about nausea and occasional vomiting, usually in the morning, as well as a skin rash on her face. Her symptoms started roughly 7 days ago. She denies fever, diarrhea, pain, and sick contacts. The facial rash began the day after she went to the beach, though she wasn't in the sun long enough to get a sunburn. The patient's last menstrual period was roughly 11 weeks ago and was normal in duration and amount of flow. Her periods usually occur once per month. The patient is otherwise in good health and takes no medications. She does not smoke or use drugs and is sexually active only with her boyfriend.

Upon further questioning, the patient mentions that she has had to go to the bathroom slightly more often than usual, though she has no dysuria. She also mentions fatigue and mild breast swelling.

Exam

T: 98.8°F   BP: 118/78   RR: 16/min.   P: 74/min.

The patient is healthy appearing and in no acute distress. Facial exam reveals scattered, macular hyperpigmentation (see figure). Heart and lung auscultation is unremarkable. The patient's breasts are full and tender, with fairly dark nipples and areolae. No breast masses are palpable. Abdominal exam is normal. Pelvic exam reveals an enlarged, somewhat soft-feeling, and globular uterus. The cervix is slightly softened, and the connection between the cervix and uterus cannot be palpated. On speculum exam, there is dark discoloration of the vaginal walls, which is also noted in the vulvar area. No vaginal discharge is identified.

Tests

Hemoglobin: 13 g/dL (normal 12–16)
White blood cell count: 6700/µL (normal 4500–11,000)
AST: 9 u/L (normal 1–27)
Urinalysis: negative for glucose, protein,
    WBCs, and bacteria

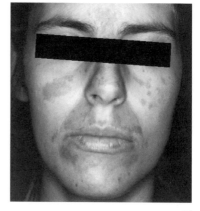

From Fitzpatrick JE, Aeling JL (eds): Dermatology Secrets. Philadelphia, Hanley & Belfus, Inc., 1996, pp 370–374;

Pregnancy

The photo shows **photodistributed macular hyperpigmentation** of the face, typical of **melasma (chloasma** or the "mask" of pregnancy).

Pathophysiology

The early signs of pregnancy are due to hormonal and other physiologic changes.

Diagnosis & Treatment

A reproductive-age female with recent onset of amenorrhea is pregnant "*until proven otherwise*." Other symptoms include **nausea and vomiting** (classically in the **morning,** thus the term "morning sickness"), **breast engorgement, weight gain, urinary frequency** (from the growing uterus pushing on the bladder), and **fatigue**.

The signs of pregnancy include **dark discoloration** of the **vulvar/vaginal walls (Chadwick's sign), nipples/areolae,** and **abdominal striae** (classically **linea nigra,** a vertical line in the midline of the lower abdomen). **Softening of the uterus** (which becomes **enlarged** and **globular**) and **cervix** is common. Softening and compressibility of the lower segment of the uterus (isthmus) can make it seem as though the neck and body of the uterus are separated during palpation (called **Hegar's sign**).

Diagnosis is usually done with a **urine β-hCG qualitative test,** though **quantitative blood tests** are available and are more sensitive. **Transvaginal ultrasound** can demonstrate evidence of pregnancy by **5 weeks** after conception. **Fetal heart tones** can be heard by **12 weeks** with a Doppler probe.

More High-Yield Facts

All sexually active, reproductive-age females are advised to take **folate** to **reduce the risk of neural tube defects**. The maximal protective effect occurs in the **first trimester,** and during much of this period, most women do not know that they are pregnant.

Don't let the fact that a patient uses birth control or has had previous sterilization prevent you from suspecting pregnancy. **No method of contraception is 100% effective,** especially when patient compliance is needed.

Obstetrics

History

A 22-year-old woman comes into your office because she recently took a home pregnancy test, and it was positive. She wants to have regular prenatal care and is not sure what is involved. Other than mild morning sickness, the patient has no health complaints. This is her first pregnancy. She has no medical problems and takes no regular medications. Her mother is a nurse and told her to ask you the following questions:

"What vitamins do I need to take, and what medications are safe?"

"What lab tests do I need?"

"How often should I come to see you?"

"Do I need to stop working and are there any other restrictions on my activities?"

Exam

T: 98.9°F   BP: 118/76   RR: 16/min.   P: 78/min.

The woman is healthy appearing and in no acute distress. Heart and lung auscultation is unremarkable. Her breasts are full and mildly tender, with no palpable breast masses. Abdominal exam is normal. Pelvic exam reveals an enlarged, somewhat soft-feeling, and globular uterus. On speculum exam, there is dark discoloration of the vaginal walls, which is also noted in the vulvar area. No vaginal discharge is identified.

Tests

Hemoglobin: 11 g/dL (normal 12–16)
Mean corpuscular volume: 80 μm/cell (normal 80–100)
Ferritin: 20 μg/L (normal 20–200)
White blood cell count: 6700/μL (normal 4500–11,000)
AST: 9 u/L (normal 1–27)
Urinalysis: negative for glucose, protein, white blood cells, and bacteria
Urine β-hCG, qualitative: positive

The patient also has **iron deficiency anemia.**

Pathophysiology

There are multiple physiologic changes in pregnancy, most of which are especially pronounced during the second or third trimester. Cardiovascular changes include slightly decreased blood pressure and **increased heart rate, stroke volume,** and, therefore, **cardiac output.** Respiratory changes include **increased tidal volume and minute ventilation** (cause the physiologic **hyperventilation/respiratory alkalosis of pregnancy**).

Lab changes include increased glomerular filtration rate (resulting in **decreased creatinine and BUN**); elevated alkaline phosphatase and **erythrocyte sedimentation rate** (worthless test in pregnancy); and **decreased hemoglobin and hematocrit** (plasma volume increases more than hemoglobin, which also increases, causing a net result of lowered H&H). Mild glycosuria and proteinuria are also normal during pregnancy. The average weight gain during pregnancy is **28 pounds**.

Diagnosis & Treatment

All reproductive-age females and pregnant women should take **folate,** and multivitamins and/or iron supplements are commonly given. Safe drugs in pregnancy include **acetaminophen** (over NSAIDs), **penicillins,** cephalosporins, **erythromycin,** diphenhydramine, docusate, and **heparin.**

Routine labs during pregnancy include: **Pap smear** (first visit), **urinalysis** (first and every visit; screens for proteinuria/pre-eclampsia and asymptomatic bacteriuria, which is treated in pregnancy due to high risk of progression to pyelonephritis), and **complete blood count.** Blood type and screen (to detect **Rh type** and any antibodies to Rh) and a syphilis screening test are also routine. Check **rubella** antibody titer in the absence of a good vaccination history. In those at risk, screen for hepatitis B, HIV, **chlamydia/gonorrhea** (age 13–25 is a risk factor!), tuberculosis, and diabetes during the first visit. A **serum alpha-fetoprotein** or "triple screen" is done routinely at **16–20 weeks,** and routine screening for **diabetes** is done at **24–28 weeks.**

At every visit, check for fetal heart tones and measure uterine size (from the symphysis pubis to the top of the fundus). Perform **ultrasound** for any **size-dates discrepancy:** the fundal height in centimeters should equal the age of the fetus in weeks between 20–35 weeks; more than 2–3 cm "off" indicates a size-dates discrepancy. Check **blood pressure** every visit (pre-eclampsia).

More High-Yield Facts

Moderate exercise, work, and sex are okay during pregnancy, but very strenuous activities should be *avoided.*

Case 26

Obstetrics

History

A 17-year-old Taiwanese girl seeks medical advice for painless, fairly heavy vaginal bleeding and excessive nausea and vomiting. She thinks she is about 16 weeks pregnant based on her last menstrual period and is concerned about the health of her baby. The patient has had no previous prenatal care and found out she was pregnant from a home pregnancy test. This is her first pregnancy. She has no significant past medical history, no history of sexually transmitted diseases, and takes no medications.

Exam

T: 98.9°F   BP: 148/92   RR: 20/min.   P: 92/min.

The girl appears anxious and mildly tachypneic. Chest and abdominal exams are unremarkable. Pelvic exam reveals an enlarged uterus, consistent with a 23-week gestational age size. No fetal heart tones are heard using a Doppler probe. No adnexal masses are appreciated. External genitalia are normal. Speculum exam shows a fresh blood clot in the vagina, as well as a rounded vesicle that resembles a grape. The patient has moderate pitting ankle edema bilaterally. An ultrasound examination reveals multiple echogenic areas alternating with cystic areas (see figure). No fetus can be visualized by either a transabdominal or transvaginal approach.

Tests

Hemoglobin: 11 g/dL (normal 12–16)
White blood cell count: 6700/μL (normal 4500–11,000)
AST: 9 u/L (normal 1–27)
Urinalysis: 3+ protein, trace glucose; negative for white blood cells and bacteria
Serum hCG, quantitative: 175,000 mIU/mL (normal pregnancy levels < 100,000)

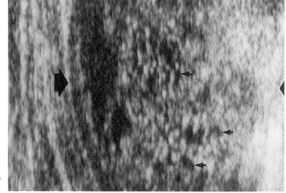

From Brant WE: Obstetric ultrasound. In Brant WE, Helms CA (eds): Fundamentals of Diagnostic Radiology, 2nd ed. Philadelphia, Lippincott, Williams & Wilkins, 1999, pp 881–906; with permission.

Gestational trophoblastic neoplasia (GTN)

GTN is also called **molar pregnancy.** The photo reveals the classic "snowstorm" appearance of a complete hydatidiform mole, the **most common type** of GTN.

Pathophysiology

In GTN, the **products of conception (the placenta)** essentially become a neoplasm. The three types of GTN in increasing order of malignancy are: benign **hydatidiform mole** (complete or incomplete), **invasive mole,** and **choriocarcinoma** (the only type that may present in women **after a normal delivery**). The cause is unknown. Patients may present during pregnancy or after any type of abortion. The tumor makes large amounts of β-hCG and **metastases** can occur. Risk factors include **Asian race, age less than 20 or more than 40,** and **previous GTN.**

Diagnosis & Treatment

Patients present with **abnormal vaginal bleeding** in the setting of current or recent pregnancy. Pregnant patients usually present in the **first or early second trimester. Hyperemesis gravidarum** or severe nausea and vomiting are common. Patients may also present with pregnancy-induced hypertension or **pre-eclampsia; hyperthyroidism** occurs only rarely and for unknown reasons.

Findings may include an **abnormally enlarged uterus** (size-dates discrepancy), tachycardia, tachypnea, **hypertension/proteinuria** (from pre-eclampsia), and **anemia.** Blood clots and/or **molar vesicles** (which **resemble grapes**) can sometimes be seen in the vagina. β-hCG levels are usually **markedly elevated** (above normal pregnancy limits). The diagnosis is generally confirmed with **ultrasound,** which may show the classic **"snowstorm"** appearance and reveal the **absence of a normal fetus.**

Treatment begins with **evacuation by dilatation and curettage** after baseline lab/radiology studies have been performed (must get **baseline quantitative β-hCG** and rule out metastases). This allows determination of the histologic type and is **curative** in the large majority of cases (85%). **Serial β-hCG levels** must then be checked to make sure the level returns to 0. If the level doesn't decline or rises, chemotherapy (**methotrexate** or actinomycin D) is given, which results in complete cure in most patients.

More High-Yield Facts

The *complete* mole karyotype is **46XX,** and **fetal tissue is absent.** The *incomplete* mole is less common, usually **69XXY,** and includes **some fetal tissue.** In both cases, all chromosomes are usually **paternal.**

If pre-eclampsia occurs in the **second trimester,** consider molar pregnancy.

Case 27

Obstetrics

History

A 22-year-old, G_1P_0, pregnant woman has come to the emergency department because of crampy lower abdominal pain and vaginal bleeding. She also thinks she may have passed a few blood clots and wonders if she has lost the baby. The patient began spotting yesterday, with the heavier bleeding starting several hours ago. Her last menstrual period was 11 weeks ago, and her periods are always regular. The patient has had no previous prenatal care and found out she was pregnant from a home pregnancy test. This is her first pregnancy. She has no significant past medical history, no history of sexually transmitted diseases, and takes no medications.

Exam

T: 98.8°F   BP: 116/74   RR: 14/min.   P: 82/min.

The woman appears anxious, but is in no acute distress. Head, chest, and abdominal exams are unremarkable, and no abdominal tenderness is evident. Pelvic exam reveals an enlarged uterus consistent with the menstrual history and no adnexal masses. Speculum exam shows the presence of vaginal blood and a few blood clots as well as a dilated cervical os.

Tests

Hemoglobin: 12 g/dL (normal 12–16)
White blood cell count: 6700/μL (normal 4500–11,000)
AST: 9 u/L (normal 1–27)
Urinalysis: negative for protein, glucose, white blood cells, and bacteria
Serum hCG, quantitative: 3000 mIU/mL (normal pregnancy levels < 100,000)
Ultrasound: endometrial canal dilatation, with probable blood in the canal;
   no intra- or extrauterine fetus visualized

Miscarriage (spontaneous abortion)

Pathophysiology

Spontaneous abortion is defined as expulsion of the fetus **before 20 weeks** or when the fetus weighs **less than 500 grams.** It is estimated to occur in **10–15%** of clinically recognizable pregnancies (many more women abort before knowing they are pregnant). About **25%** of women have first trimester **bleeding,** and 50% of these women end up having a miscarriage.

There are several abortion terms, all of which imply that the event occurs prior to 20 weeks. **Threatened** abortion is vaginal bleeding with a closed cervix. **Inevitable** abortion is vaginal bleeding, crampy abdominal pain, and a partially dilated cervix. **Incomplete** abortion is vaginal bleeding, abdominal pain, cervical dilatation, and passage of fetal tissue. **Completed** abortion implies that all products of conception have been expelled, the bleeding has stopped, and the cervical os is closed. **Missed** abortion is when a fetus dies, but remains in the uterus for several weeks without being expelled. **Recurrent** abortion is two or three successive spontaneous abortions and often implies a specific underlying disorder.

Diagnosis & Treatment

As described above, women present with **vaginal bleeding** before 20 weeks' gestation (most in the first trimester) and may have **crampy abdominal pain.**

Exam may reveal an open or closed **cervical os** and blood, **blood clots,** and/or products of conception in the vagina. The quantitative **β-hCG** is often in the low-normal or below-normal range for the gestational age. Pelvic **ultrasound** is performed on **all women** to examine the status of the pregnancy. Absence of evidence for an intrauterine pregnancy after 5 weeks' gestation (assuming the dates are accurate) generally indicates **fetal loss.**

Treatment for threatened abortion is **supportive** care and routine follow-up only. **Pelvic rest** is advised (no sex). Treatment for other types of abortion includes IV fluids, **Rh immune globulin** (RhoGAM) for Rh-negative moms, and **counseling.** Expectant management (observation, monitoring with serial β-hCG levels) can be used for completed abortions. For incomplete and inevitable abortions, **dilatation and curettage** or **vacuum suction** are recommended, especially if bleeding is excessive, vital signs are unstable, or infected tissue is present in the uterine cavity. In the future, expectant or **medical** (e.g., prostaglandin) treatment may become an acceptable option for uncomplicated inevitable or incomplete abortions.

More High-Yield Facts

The most common identifiable cause of spontaneous abortion is thought to be **fetal chromosomal abnormalities** (usually some form of **trisomy**).

Obstetrics

History

A 16-year-old, pregnant, black girl complains of headache and blurry vision that began yesterday, and swelling in her face, hands, and feet that began a week ago. She is G_1P_0, carrying twins, and 31 weeks pregnant by dates. The patient has missed her last four routine prenatal appointments due to lack of transportation. The pregnancy appeared to be progressing normally the last time you saw her, and there were no abnormal physical exam or laboratory findings. The patient has no significant past medical history and takes no regular medications.

Exam

T: 98.9°F   BP: 166/94   RR: 18/min.   P: 92/min.

The patient's face is puffy and edematous. Her visual acuity is grossly diminished. Chest and abdominal exams are unremarkable. Pelvic exam reveals no obvious abnormalities and, two sets of fetal heart tones can be heard. There is marked (3–4+) edema in both the hands and feet.

Tests

Hemoglobin: 16 g/dL (normal 12–16)
White blood cell count: 6700/μL (normal 4500–11,000)
Platelet count: 155,000/μL (normal 150,000–400,000)
AST: 39 u/L (normal 1–27)
ALT: 36 u/L (normal 1–21)
Creatinine: 0.6 mg/dL (normal 0.6–1.5)
Urinalysis: 4+ proteinuria, 1+ glucose; negative for white blood cells and
   bacteria

Pre-eclampsia, severe

Pathophysiology

Pregnancy-induced hypertension (PIH) includes isolated hypertension, pre-eclampsia, and eclampsia. The cause is unknown. Risk factors include **chronic renal disease, pre-existing hypertension, family or personal history of PIH, multiple gestation pregnancy, nulliparity, extremes of reproductive age, diabetes, and black race.**

Pre-eclampsia and eclampsia are important because they cause uteroplacental insufficiency, intrauterine growth retardation, and **increased fetal and maternal morbidity and mortality.** Eclampsia is pre-eclampsia plus seizures.

Diagnosis & Treatment

Classic complaints occur in a **young female** during the **third trimester** of her **first pregnancy** and include face, hand, and/or leg **swelling; decreased urine output; headaches; visual disturbances; altered mental status;** and epigastric or right upper quadrant (RUQ) **abdominal pain.**

The classic triad of findings includes **hypertension** (> 140/90 or an increase of > 30 mmHg systolic or 15 mmHg diastolic from baseline), **proteinuria** (2+ or more on urinalysis), and face, hand, and severe ankle **edema** (mild ankle edema is normal in pregnancy). Hypertension plus proteinuria is pre-eclampsia *"until proven otherwise."* Rapid **weight gain** from edema may be noted. Patients may develop (rarely) the **HELLP syndrome** (h̲emolysis, e̲levated l̲iver enzymes, and l̲ow p̲latelets, often accompanied by RUQ pain). **Oliguria** and hyperuricemia may also be seen.

Definitive treatment is **delivery after maternal stabilization** (don't perform a c-section if the mother is in the middle of a seizure). Those with *mild disease*—defined as BP < 160/110, mild to moderate proteinuria (1–2+), no HELLP findings, and no symptoms besides edema—can be treated medically on an inpatient basis with **BP control** (using hydralazine or labetalol) and **observation.** *In all other cases,* **labor induction or c-section** is indicated. **Magnesium sulfate** is used initially to control seizures in those with eclampsia; it also helps control BP. If magnesium is given, watch for **toxicity,** which can cause **decreased deep tendon reflexes,** hypotension, and **respiratory depression.** If this occurs, *stop* the infusion.

More High-Yield Facts

PIH is one of the leading causes of **maternal mortality** (along with pulmonary embolism and hemorrhage). PIH does *not* increase the risk of hypertension later in life.

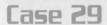

Case 29

Obstetrics

History

A 37-year-old, G_2P_0 woman presents for a routine prenatal visit. She is 31 weeks pregnant by dates and by ultrasound performed in the mid-first trimester for an episode of threatened abortion. Since then, the pregnancy has progressed normally, though the patient has not been to see you for 2 months, missing her last two appointments due to "an extremely busy work schedule." The patient complains of fatigue, mentioning that she is under tremendous stress at work and has been unable to cut back on her smoking and drinking and, in fact, has increased her consumption of both alcohol and cigarettes since the last time she saw you. She also admits that her nutrition consists primarily of fast food take-out meals.

The patient's past medical history is significant only for hypertension, for which the patient takes labetalol. Her baseline blood pressure runs in the 140–160/85–95 range, and medication compliance has been a problem. Her first pregnancy ended in a miscarriage at 10 weeks, after an all-night cocaine binge. She denies current cocaine use.

Exam

T: 98.6°F   BP: 142/90   RR: 16/min.   P: 82/min.

The patient is in no acute distress. Head, neck, chest, and abdominal exams are unremarkable. The patient's fingers are nicotine stained. The fundal height is measured at 25 cm. Normal fetal heart tones are heard. Pelvic exam is unremarkable. No significant edema is noted.

Tests

Hemoglobin: 10 g/dL (normal 12–16)
White blood cell count: 6700/μL (normal 4500–11,000)
Creatinine: 0.6 mg/dL (normal 0.6–1.5)
Urinalysis: trace proteinuria and glycosuria; negative for white blood cells and bacteria
Ultrasound: fetal biparietal diameter and head circumference 10th percentile for age; abdominal circumference and femur length below 5th percentile; mild oligohydramnios; no fetal anomalies detected

Intrauterine growth retardation (IUGR)

In this case, IUGR is likely secondary to maternal and possibly placental factors.

Pathophysiology

IUGR is defined as fetal size less than the 10th percentile for gestational age. Therefore, **accurate dating** is important before diagnosing IUGR. Causes can be divided into three main categories: **maternal** (nutrition, smoking/alcohol/drug use, cardiac or pulmonary disease, stress, anemia, antiphospholipid syndrome, prior IUGR), **placental** (placental insufficiency from maternal hypertension, renal disease, pregnancy-induced hypertension), and **fetal** (congenital anomalies, intrauterine infections). IUGR infants have a **higher risk of perinatal morbidity and mortality,** including fetal anomalies, neurodevelopmental delays or retardation, prenatal or intrapartum asphyxia, neonatal hypoglycemia, and meconium aspiration.

Diagnosis & Treatment

Patients usually have no complaints, but may have a history of one or more **maternal risk factors** discussed above.

Exam may reveal a **size-dates discrepancy**, which occurs when the number of centimeters for fundal height is $2+$ cm less than the number of gestational weeks. Any size-dates discrepancy is an indication for **ultrasound** examination, which will reveal growth parameters **< 10th percentile for age** when IUGR is present. The main growth parameters in clinical use are the **biparietal diameter, head circumference, abdominal circumference**, and **femur length**. **Oligohydramnios** is common.

IUGR pregnancies are considered to be **high risk.** Treatment is directed at any **correctable factors** (e.g., drug/alcohol/tobacco use, anemia). Weekly **biophysical profile testing** (BPP) is indicated in the 3rd trimester, with an **oxytocin stress test** used if the BPP is unfavorable. **Induced delivery** or **cesarean section** is often recommended if the BPP or stress test is abnormal, especially if fetal lung maturity is adequate (lecithin:sphingomyelin ratio > 2 in amniotic fluid obtained by amniocentesis).

More High-Yield Facts

Low-dose aspirin may help prevent IUGR in women with the antiphospholipid antibody syndrome.

IUGR can be **symmetric** (whole body affected, usually from fetal anomalies or infections) or **asymmetric** (the **head size is normal,** due to maternal or placental factors). Asymmetric IUGR is more common.

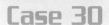

Case 30

Obstetrics

History

A 22-year-old woman has come to the emergency department because of severe abdominal pain and vaginal bleeding. She says the pain started suddenly 2 hours ago and nearly caused her to pass out. She still feels somewhat light-headed. The patient also feels nauseous and vomited once when the pain first started. Her last menstrual period was 7–8 weeks ago, though her periods usually occur very regularly every 4 weeks. Past medical history is remarkable only for two episodes of chlamydia, one of which required hospitalization according to the patient because the infection was "really bad."

The patient is sexually active and uses condoms regularly. She takes no regular medications and has never been pregnant.

Exam

T: 99.5°F   BP: 102/62   RR: 24/min.   P: 122/min.

The patient looks pale, is diaphoretic, has tachypnea, and becomes dizzy when she tries to stand up. Her skin is cold and clammy. Chest exam reveals clear lungs and tachycardia. Her pulse is weak, and capillary refill is delayed. Abdominal exam reveals tenderness and voluntary guarding throughout the abdomen, most severe in the left lower quadrant, with mild rebound tenderness. Bowel sounds are decreased. Pelvic exam reveals a left adnexal mass and tenderness. Speculum exam shows fresh blood in the vagina, but no other abnormalities.

Tests

Hemoglobin: 10 g/dL (normal 12–16)
White blood cell count: 11,700/μL (normal 4500–11,000)
Creatinine: 0.8 mg/dL (normal 0.6–1.5)
BUN: 25 mg/dL (normal 8–25)
Urinalysis: negative for protein, glucose, white blood cells, and bacteria; high specific gravity
Urine β-hCG, qualitative: positive

Ectopic pregnancy with rupture

Pathophysiology

Most ectopic pregnancies occur in the **fallopian tubes** (95%), though ovarian and even abdominal pregnancies are possible. Risk factors for developing an ectopic pregnancy include **pelvic inflammatory disease/salpingitis,** use of an **intrauterine device, prior ectopic pregnancy,** history of **tubal surgery, pelvic adhesions, endometriosis,** and **intrauterine diethylstilbestrol exposure.** Ectopic pregnancies are now the fourth leading cause of maternal mortality and the **leading cause of maternal death in the first trimester.**

Tubal ectopic pregnancies generally either **abort** or **rupture** in the first trimester if an early diagnosis is not made.

Diagnosis & Treatment

The classic triad of symptoms in ectopic pregnancy is **amenorrhea, vaginal bleeding, and abdominal pain. Nausea** and **vomiting** are fairly common. A history of one or more **risk factors** (as discussed above) may also be present. Lightheadedness/dizziness, syncope, and/or altered mental status are ominous findings that generally indicate **rupture.**

Physical exam reveals **abdominal tenderness,** which generally includes peritoneal signs only if rupture occurs. Signs of **hypovolemia and shock** (tachycardia, tachypnea, hypotension, orthostasis, delayed capillary refill) also usually indicate rupture and internal hemorrhage. An **adnexal mass** may be present, and can represent the ectopic pregnancy or a **corpus luteum cyst.** Low-grade **fever** may be present, especially with rupture. **The β-hCG is always positive.**

In stable patients, pelvic **ultrasound** is used to confirm the diagnosis (successful in most cases). **Culdocentesis** is rarely used anymore, but may reveal blood in the cul-de-sac. Unstable patients (such as the one in this case) should proceed **directly to laparotomy**/laparoscopy for diagnosis and treatment. Supportive management for shock (e.g., IV fluids and/or blood transfusion) is also important. Laparotomy/ laparoscopy is the treatment of choice once the diagnosis is confirmed in stable patients. **Tube-sparing surgery** may be possible; otherwise, salpingectomy is used. Give **Rh immune globulin** to Rh-negative women.

More High-Yield Facts

Medical management of small tubal pregnancies with **methotrexate** (to induce abortion) is an option for small (< 3 cm) tubal pregnancies, if the patient is compliant and strongly desires this option.

Case 31

Obstetrics

History

A 37-year-old G_2P_1 woman presents to the emergency department claiming that she is in labor. She says that she is in her 38th week of pregnancy and she began having contractions several hours ago that are now roughly 15 minutes apart and regular. Her first child was delivered by cesarean section 2 years ago because the baby "wasn't doing well" at the time of labor.

Exam

T: 98.5°F   BP: 122/84   RR: 18/min.   P: 82/min.

The patient is currently in no acute distress. Chest exam is unremarkable. Abdominal exam reveals a gravid uterus consistent with a term gestation. Fetal heart tones are normal. Palpation of the fetus reveals a vertex presentation. Pelvic exam shows that the cervix is dilated 2 cm and 30% effaced. The woman is admitted, and fetal heart and uterine contraction pattern monitoring is established. A particular pattern persists for 40 minutes (see figure). During this time, the mother complains that her contractions are becoming stronger. The fetal scalp pH is 6.9 (normal 7.26–7.42).

Tests

Hemoglobin: 13 g/dL (normal 12–16)   WBCs: 7700/µL (normal 4500–11,000)
Urinalysis: trace glucose; negative for protein, white blood cells, and bacteria

Fetal Heart Rate (beats per minute)

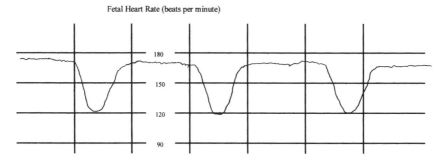

Uterine contraction pattern (pressure measured in mmHg)

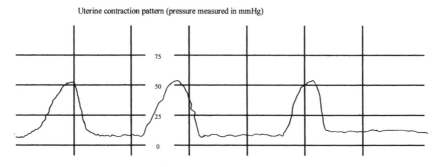

Fetal distress

In this case, fetal distress is likely due to uteroplacental insufficiency. The fetal heart strip demonstrates repeated late decelerations.

Pathophysiology

Intrapartum fetal monitoring is somewhat controversial, but almost universal in labor and delivery units in the U.S. Three primary patterns of fetal heart **decelerations** (heart rate decreases at least 15 bpm below baseline) are early, variable, and late. **Early** decelerations are due to **head compression** and are considered **normal.** The nadir (lowest point) of fetal heart rate occurs at the **same time** as the peak of the uterine contraction. **Variable** decelerations are thought to be due to transient **umbilical cord compression** and have **no relation** to the uterine contraction pattern.

Late decelerations are thought to be due to **uteroplacental insufficiency** and are **worrisome** if they persist (the more the fetal heart rate declines, the more worrisome the pattern is). The nadir of the fetal heart rate occurs just *after* the peak of the uterine contraction. **Lack of beat-to-beat variability** (normal heart rate changes that give a somewhat wavy appearance to the baseline heart rate) is considered another possible sign of fetal distress. **Prolonged** and **marked** fetal **bradycardia** or **tachycardia** (normal heart rate is 120–160) is also worrisome.

Diagnosis & Treatment

The mother is often **asymptomatic,** but may have **hypotension, hypoxia,** or **painful uterine contractions** (especially in the setting of oxytocin administration) in some cases. Many cases of fetal distress occur in the setting of a **high-risk pregnancy.**

A **persistent pattern** of **late or variable decelerations** on fetal heart monitoring should first be managed by having the mom lay in a **left lateral position** and giving supplemental **oxygen.** Oxytocin should be *stopped* if it is being administered, and **IV fluids** given, especially in the setting of maternal **hypotension.** If either pattern persists for more than **30 minutes** despite these measures, check the **fetal scalp pH.** If the pH is **< 7.2** or fetal blood cannot be sampled due to lack of cervical dilatation, c-section is usually indicated. If the fetal pH is > 7.2, continued observation is advisable.

More High-Yield Facts

Fetal heart monitoring is controversial because randomized trials **failed to demonstrate** any true **benefit.** However, it is commonly used, especially in high-risk pregnancies, and the basic patterns are fair game for the boards.

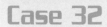

Case 32

Obstetrics

History

A 38-year-old, G_6P_5, pregnant woman is in the emergency department because of painless, bright red, vaginal bleeding that began 2 hours ago. She is currently at 33 weeks' gestation. The patient denies uterine contractions and has had no previous problems during this pregnancy. She denies tobacco, drug, and alcohol use and has not had recent sex or trauma. She has no history of a bleeding disorder. All five of her children are currently healthy, though three of them were delivered by cesarean section for a "placenta in the wrong place."

Exam

T: 98.5°F   BP: 126/80   RR: 18/min.   P: 82/min.

The patient is currently in no acute distress. Chest exam is unremarkable. Abdominal exam reveals a gravid uterus without tenderness. Fetal heart tones are present and indicate mild fetal tachycardia. A small amount of bright red blood is noted at the introitus. No peripheral edema is apparent.

Tests

Hemoglobin: 13 g/dL (normal 12–16)
White blood cell count: 7700/μL (normal 4500–11,000)
Creatinine: 0.8 mg/dL (normal 0.6–1.5)
BUN: 8 mg/dL (normal 8–25)
Urinalysis: negative for protein, glucose, white blood cells, and bacteria
Urine drug screen: negative

Third-trimester bleeding

In this case, placenta previa is the most likely cause.

Pathophysiology

Third-trimester bleeding is considered an obstetric **emergency** and occurs in roughly 5% of pregnancies. There are multiple causes, including **placenta previa, abruptio placentae, uterine rupture, fetal vessel rupture/vasa previa, cervical** or **vaginal lesions,** and **bleeding disorders.** Being able to distinguish between these causes is high-yield for the boards.

Placenta previa occurs when the placenta covers the internal **cervical os** (can be complete or partial). Risk factors include **increasing maternal age, multiparity, multiple gestation, prior placenta previa,** and **prior uterine surgery/c-section.**

Diagnosis & Treatment

Patients with previa classically present with **painless, bright red vaginal bleeding** in the third trimester. They usually are in **no distress** and are *not* having contractions. One or more **risk factors** discussed above may be present.

In the presence of third-trimester bleeding, a **pelvic exam is contraindicated until ultrasound has been performed to rule out a placenta previa,** as disturbance of the placenta in this setting can cause worsening hemorrhage and turn an urgent situation into a critical one. All women with third-trimester bleeding should receive **IV fluids** (and/or blood transfusions for severe hemorrhage) and **supplemental oxygen.** Fetal and maternal **monitoring** are also indicated. Check a **complete blood count, coagulation profiles,** and a **urine drug screen** if there is any suspicion. After a partial physical exam, perform an ultrasound to rule out placenta previa. If the ultrasound is negative for previa, do a careful speculum and pelvic exam to look for other causes of bleeding and to check the cervix.

If placenta previa is noted on ultrasound, treatment is prompt **cesarean section** if the woman is at **term** or there is **fetal distress.** Hospital admission and **observation with tocolysis** can be performed for **preterm** mothers **if mom and baby are stable** and **the bleeding stops** on its own. Elective c-section will eventually be required, as **vaginal delivery is contraindicated** with placenta previa.

More High-Yield Facts

Some form of previa or low-lying placenta (not technically previa, but the placenta implants in the lower uterine segment) occurs in at least one-third of second-trimester pregnancies. At least **90%** of these placentas migrate upward during continued uterine growth and **reach "normal" position** by the time of delivery. If previa is noted in the second trimester, do follow-up ultrasound early in the third trimester to reassess the placenta.

Case 33

Obstetrics

History

A 17-year-old, G_1P_0, white female, currently at 10 weeks gestation by last menstrual period, is suffering severe, constant nausea and vomiting. She has been unable to keep down any food or liquids for the past 4 days, so her mother brought her to the emergency department. The patient denies fever, sick contacts, diarrhea, jaundice, melena, hematemesis, dysuria, and abdominal pain. She has had trouble sleeping because of her symptoms. The patient does not smoke, drink alcohol, or use drugs and has no history of eating disorders. She claims weight loss of 9 pounds since becoming pregnant because of her nausea and vomiting; she now weighs 115 pounds. The patient's mother takes you aside and mentions that her daughter is "rather immature and histrionic."

Exam

T: 98.7°F   BP: 116/74   RR: 18/min.   P: 82/min.

The patient looks dehydrated and has a dry, coated tongue. She has decreased skin turgor. Chest and abdominal exams are unremarkable and reveal no tenderness. Pelvic exam reveals an appropriately enlarged uterus with no adnexal masses. Speculum exam is unremarkable. No peripheral edema is noted.

Tests

Hemoglobin: 12 g/dL (normal 12–16)
White blood cell count: 7700/µL (normal 4500–11,000)
Sodium: 135 meq/L (normal 135–145)
Chloride: 93 mmol/L (normal 100–108)
Potassium: 3.3 meq/L (normal 3.5–5)
CO_2: 32 meq/L (normal 24–30)
Creatinine: 0.8 mg/dL (normal 0.6–1.5)
BUN: 20 mg/dL (normal 8–25)
AST: 25 u/L (normal 7–27)
ALT: 19 u/L (normal 1–21)
β-hCG, quantitative: elevated (appropriate for gestational age)
TSH: 1.9 µU/mL (normal 0.5–5)
Lipase: 8 u/dL (normal 4–24)
Serum ketones: positive (1+)
Urinalysis: 2+ ketones; negative for protein, glucose, white blood cells, and
    bacteria
Urine drug screen: negative
Glucose: 90 mg/dl (normal < 200)

Pathophysiology

Nausea and vomiting ("morning sickness") are extremely common during pregnancy and are thought to be due to **hormonal changes,** including elevation of β-hCG and estrogen levels. Hyperemesis gravidarum occurs in roughly **1%** of pregnancies, with symptoms that become intractable and may result in dehydration and electrolyte disturbances requiring hospitalization and, rarely, parenteral nutrition.

The reason some women develop this condition is unknown. The risk for hyperemesis is increased with **white race, age < 25,** and the **first pregnancy. Psychological factors** are classically thought to play a role (e.g., hysterical, immature, or dependent personalities), but controlled studies have *not* proved this.

Diagnosis & Treatment

Hyperemesis generally presents in the **first trimester,** but may last well into the second trimester. Patients report **intractable nausea and vomiting** that prevents keeping down any solids or liquids. Symptoms may **interfere with sleep** and cause at least a **5% weight loss.**

Findings include signs of **dehydration** (dry mucous membranes, coated tongue, poor skin turgor, elevated BUN:creatinine ratio), **weight loss, ketonuria** and **ketonemia,** and **electrolyte disturbances** (hyponatremia, hypokalemia, and hypochloremic metabolic alkalosis). In severe cases, liver or renal function tests may be abnormal. The diagnosis is made **clinically. Ultrasound** is generally performed to assess the fetus and rule out a molar pregnancy.

Treatment is **IV fluids** and **correction of any electrolyte abnormalities** on an inpatient basis. Patients are encouraged to eat **small, non-spicy, frequent meals. Antiemetic drugs** (diphenhydramine, prochlorperazine) may be needed (fairly safe). Psychological **counseling** is advised to help the patient deal with the frustration the disorder causes and help identify any correctable life stressors. **Parenteral nutrition** is sometimes required.

More High-Yield Facts

Hyperemesis gravidarum is a **diagnosis of exclusion,** and serious conditions that cause nausea and vomiting, such as pyelonephritis, pancreatitis, or cholecystitis, must be ruled out in the appropriate setting.

A **molar pregnancy** can present as hyperemesis gravidarum. It is effectively ruled out with a normal ultrasound and β-hCG level.

Obstetrics

History

A 19-year-old, G_1P_1 woman who is 3 weeks postpartum is troubled by a painful right breast that began bothering her last night. She has also experienced fever, malaise, and mild chills for the past 2 days. The patient is currently breast-feeding, which she says is now painful in her right breast. Several days prior to her symptoms, a painful crack developed in her right nipple; she kept hoping it would go away, but it didn't. Her child is healthy, was delivered vaginally at term without complications, and has not been sick. The patient denies any recent sick contacts, and her only significant pat medical history is obesity. She takes no medications and does not smoke or drink alcohol.

Exam

T: 102.8°F   BP: 136/84   RR: 16/min.   P: 84/min.

The patient is obese, but in no acute distress. Chest exam reveals erythema, tenderness, and induration of the entire medial inferior aspect of the right breast. No underlying mass or fluctuance is identified, but a slightly macerated fissure is noted in the right nipple. The left breast is normal, as is the rest of the examination. No skin rash is identified.

Tests

Hemoglobin: 12 g/dL (normal 12–16)
White blood cell count: 11,900/μL (normal 4500–11,000)
Platelet count: 200,000/μL (normal 150,000–400,000)
AST: 15 u/L (normal 7–27)
Urinalysis: negative for protein, glucose, white blood cells, and bacteria

Pathophysiology

Mastitis is an uncommon complication of breast-feeding. The most common etiology is *Staphylococcus aureus* infection. The bacteria gain entry through the skin due to a cracked, fissured, or irritated nipple, and are thought to originate from the **infant's oropharynx.**

Diagnosis & Treatment

Most women present **2 to 4 weeks postpartum. Fever** (which may be high), **chills,** and **malaise** are common. A focal area of **pain** and **redness** is present in the involved breast. The infant is usually **healthy,** as the bacteria are from his/her normal flora. Women may also relate a history of a prior crack or irritation in their nipple.

Exam reveals fever and a **focal area** of breast **erythema, tenderness,** and **induration.** In 10% of cases, underlying **fluctuance** may be present, which indicates the development of an **abscess.**

Treatment includes **culture** of the breast milk from the affected side and empiric treatment with **antibiotics** to cover *S. aureus* (e.g., **dicloxacillin, cefazolin**). Milk should **continue** to be expressed from the breast, either by continued nursing or a breast pump if nursing is too painful. **Analgesics** and **local moist-heat applications** are important supportive measures. If an abscess develops, **surgical incision and drainage** are advisable, and nursing should be **discontinued** until healing has occurred.

If the nipples become markedly irritated, cracked, or fissured, aggressive management to **prevent** mastitis is indicated. This includes **temporary cessation** of breast-feeding (with manual breast milk expression to maintain flow and prevent discomfort), use of a **nipple shield,** and application of an appropriate breast cream or ointment.

More High-Yield Facts

Breast-feeding is recommended for **financial** reasons, mother-infant bonding, and **fetal health benefits** (**IgA** secreted in breast milk provides passive immunization). If a mom chooses not to breast-feed, treatment can be offered to reduce discomfort and suppress lactation. **Tight-fitting bras, ice packs,** and **analgesics** can be used, as well as **bromocriptine** (a dopamine agonist that suppresses prolactin levels and inhibits lactation). Manual expression of milk can make things *worse.* If these measures aren't used, women may present with severe, **bilateral** breast engorgement and redness, which shouldn't be confused with bacterial mastitis.

Case 35

Obstetrics

History

A 27-year-old woman presents to the clinic with her husband of 7 years after a home pregnancy test revealed that she was pregnant. She has been pregnant twice before. The first pregnancy was 2 years ago, but the patient had an elective abortion that was complicated by fairly heavy bleeding requiring overnight hospitalization. The second pregnancy was 9 months ago and ended in a miscarriage at 8 weeks. The patient currently has no complaints, desires to have the child, and says her last menstrual period was 8 weeks ago. Her past medical history is otherwise noncontributory and she takes no medications other than a daily multivitamin. She does not smoke, drink alcohol, or use drugs.

She mentions to you that her previous doctor told her she may have a problem in the future because of her blood type and asks you to check both her and her husband's blood type to see if there is a problem.

Exam

T: 98.6°F   BP: 116/78   RR: 14/min.   P: 66/min.

The patient is athletic appearing and in no acute distress. Head, neck, chest, and abdominal exams are unremarkable. Pelvic exam reveals a mildly enlarged, smooth, globular uterus, consistent with early pregnancy. External genitalia are normal, as is a speculum exam.

Tests

Hemoglobin: 15 g/dL (normal 12–16)
White blood cell count: 6100/μL (normal 4500–11,000)
Platelet count: 200,000/μL (normal 150,000–400,000)
AST: 15 u/L (normal 7–27)
Urinalysis: negative for protein, glucose, white blood cells, and bacteria
Rapid plasmin reagin for syphilis screening: negative
Blood type: O
Rhesus antigen: negative

Husband's blood type: A
Husband's rhesus antigen: positive

Pathophysiology

The rhesus antigen on blood cells may be present (Rh+) or absent (Rh–) in normal persons. In the U.S., **15%** of whites are Rh–. If a woman who is Rh– is exposed to Rh+ blood (from fetal blood crossing the placenta or prior blood transfusion), she may form antibodies against the Rh antigen. IgG anti-Rh antibodies can cross the placenta and cause **hemolysis, anemia, hyperbilirubinemia,** and even death (**fetal hydrops**) in an Rh+ fetus.

The mother has to be **Rh–** and the father **Rh+** (or, often, the father's blood type is unknown) for the fetus to have a chance of being Rh+. Because a first exposure is needed to produce "sensitization," the first pregnancy is often *not affected,* but without prophylactic treatment, future pregnancies may develop serious complications. Other blood cell antigens (e.g., the **Kell** antigen) can also cause this problem (though rarely).

Diagnosis & Treatment

In current practice, potential cases of Rh incompatibility are usually identified with **routine screening** of Rh status at the **first prenatal visit.** If mom is Rh– and dad is Rh+ (or unknown), order an Rh antibody titer or **indirect Coombs test** (less specific, but detects other minor antigens that may cause problems). If Rh antibodies are present, *sensitization has already occurred.* Close monitoring until term is required, with periodic amniotic fluid **spectrophotometry** and **ultrasound** to detect complications. Early delivery, intrauterine fetal transfusion, and/or **phenobarbital** to hasten fetal liver bilirubin breakdown (prevents **kernicterus**) may be needed. Rh immune globulin (RhoGAM) *won't work* in these cases (too late).

If mom is Rh– but has no antibodies, your job is to prevent them from developing. In addition to rechecking for antibody development in the **third trimester,** give RhoGAM at **28 weeks** and within **72 hours** after delivery. RhoGAM attaches to the fetal red blood cells and prevents a maternal immune response by covering up the antigen. In addition, give RhoGAM for any event that **increases the risk of fetomaternal hemorrhage** (e.g., abortion, stillbirth, ectopic pregnancy, amniocentesis, chorionic villus sampling, antepartum bleeding). Giving RhoGAM is an example of **primary prevention.**

More High-Yield Facts

The **Kleihauer-Betke** maternal blood test can quantify the amount of fetomaternal hemorrhage. This is sometimes useful to calculate a dose of RhoGAM.

Obstetrics

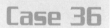

History

A 24-year-old, G_4P_0, pregnant woman complains of vaginal discharge and dysuria. Her symptoms started 2 weeks ago. She has not had any routine prenatal care, but reports no problems with the pregnancy and thinks she is about 4 or 5 months pregnant. The woman has had three prior elective abortions, but says she wants to keep her current child. She has a prior history of treated sexually transmitted diseases and is sexually active with multiple partners. She is single and is not sure which of her partners is the father of the child. The patient takes no medications and is a recovered cocaine addict.

Exam

T: 98.6°F   BP: 126/82   RR: 16/min.   P: 86/min.

The patient is obviously pregnant, but in no acute distress. Head, neck, and chest exams are unremarkable. Abdominal exam reveals a gravid uterus with normal bowel sounds. The fundal height is consistent with a 20-week gestation. There are no adnexal masses and cervical os is closed on pelvic exam. Speculum exam shows a mucopurulent discharge and a mildly erythematous cervix. Under a microscope, numerous white blood cells are evident in the discharge, but no clue cells, intracellular diplococci, yeast, or trichomonads are seen. A rapid chlamydial antigen detection test is positive. No external genitalia lesions are seen.

Tests

Hemoglobin: 12 g/dL (normal 12–16)
White blood cell count: 6100/μL (normal 4500–11,000)
AST: 15 u/L (normal 7–27)
HIV ELISA test: positive
Rapid plasmin reagin for syphilis screening: negative
Urinalysis: negative for protein, glucose, white blood cells and bacteria.

Pregnancy complicated by HIV and *Chlamydia trachomatis*

Pathophysiology

Human immunodeficiency virus (HIV) and chlamydia are both sexually transmitted diseases (STDs) that can complicate pregnancy. Both infections are more commonly seen in **single, promiscuous, nonwhite women under age 25** from **urban** areas. Both can be transmitted to the fetus and therefore require treatment to reduce this risk. Maternal chlamydial infection increases the risk of **prematurity,** preterm premature rupture of the membranes (**PPROM**), and postpartum **endometritis,** as well as neonatal **conjunctivitis,** otitis media, and **pneumonia.** HIV in children markedly reduces life span and quality of life.

Diagnosis & Treatment

HIV testing should be offered to **all women** (consent is required). Screening for all other STDs (especially chlamydia, gonorrhea, hepatitis B, and syphilis) should be done at the **first prenatal visit,** especially in single women **under age 25.** Treatment for chlamydia during pregnancy is **erythromycin, amoxicillin,** or azithromycin (avoid doxycycline and quinolones).

HIV treatment during *and* after pregnancy results in at least a 65% **reduction** in fetal transmission (25% to 8% in one classic study). Moms should be given **AZT** (with or without other antiretrovirals—an evolving area) in the second and third trimester (sooner if mom has symptomatic HIV) and during the intrapartum period (intravenous AZT). The baby should be given AZT for the **first 6 weeks** of life. If women present during labor without prior prenatal care, antiretroviral therapy should be started immediately, as this still reduces transmission significantly. Elective (pre-planned) **cesarean section** is also currently thought to reduce the risk of HIV transmission. **Breast-feeding is contraindicated.**

In general, the mother's HIV infection should be treated and managed **as if she weren't pregnant** (e.g., give *Pneumocystis* prophylaxis if the CD_4 count is below 200; treat opportunistic infections if they occur; monitor viral load and CD_4 counts). Involve an expert in HIV care, who can help select therapies with the **least teratogenic** potential.

More High-Yield Facts

Testing in newborns is done with a **polymerase chain reaction test** to detect viral DNA directly, as **maternal antibodies** that cross the placenta will give **false positives** with the ELISA test. Follow-up testing at 2 and 6 months is needed to confirm or exclude the diagnosis.

Obstetrics

History

A 29-year-old, G_5P_4, pregnant woman presents to the emergency department with a chief complaint of vaginal bleeding and lower abdominal pain. The patient believes these symptoms are due to contractions. She thinks she is about 9 months pregnant, but has had no prenatal care. Her symptoms began suddenly 3 hours ago. The patient has had four prior vaginal deliveries without complications. Past medical history is remarkable for hypertension and drug and tobacco abuse. The patient denies current drug use and takes no regular medication. She says she ran out of her blood pressure medicine a few weeks ago and didn't have the money to get the prescription refilled.

Exam

T: 98.6°F   BP: 176/98   RR: 20/min.   P: 106/min.

The patient is agitated and in moderate distress. She is obviously pregnant and mildly diaphoretic. Her pupils are markedly dilated, but reactive and symmetric. The fingers of her right hand are nicotine stained. Chest exam reveals clear lungs and tachycardia without murmurs. Abdominal exam reveals normal bowel sounds and a tender gravid uterus, with increased tone and frequent contractions. The size of the uterus is consistent with a term pregnancy. Auscultation of fetal heart tones reveals fetal tachycardia with a rate of 190. Dark red blood is noted at the introitus.

Tests

Hemoglobin: 12 g/dL (normal 12–16)
White blood cell count: 9100/μL (normal 4500–11,000)
Platelet count: 420,000/μL (normal 150,000–400,000)
AST: 15 u/L (normal 7–27)
Urinalysis: negative for protein, glucose, white blood cells, and bacteria
Urine drug screen: positive for cocaine
Ultrasound exam: pending

Pathophysiology

Placental abruption occurs when the placenta **prematurely detaches,** which can result in **hemorrhage.** Risk factors for abruption include maternal **hypertension** (most important risk factor and may be pre-existing or pregnancy-induced), **pre-eclampsia, polyhydramnios, cocaine and tobacco abuse, increasing parity, prior abruption,** and **preterm premature rupture of the membranes.**

The health of the mother (hypotension, disseminated intravascular coagulation) and baby (hypoxia, anemia, death) are threatened by this condition.

Diagnosis & Treatment

Classic symptoms are **vaginal bleeding** and **lower abdominal, pelvic, or uterine pain.** The pain is generally due to uterine irritation and contractions. Many women have one or more risk factors discussed above.

As with all cases of third-trimester bleeding, perform type and crossmatch, give IV fluids (and/or blood products) and oxygen, and set up maternal and fetal monitoring. An **ultrasound must be done before pelvic exam** to rule out placenta previa. Ultrasound is fairly **insensitive** in detecting abruption.

Classic findings for abruption are **vaginal bleeding** (the blood is usually **dark red** or "port-wine" colored) and **uterine tenderness** with **increased tone** and **hyperactivity** (i.e., frequent contractions). Maternal **hypotension** or **fetal distress** (e.g., fetal tachycardia) may be present with increasing amounts of blood loss.

If mom and baby are stable and the pregnancy is term, **vaginal delivery** is generally preferred (induction of delivery with oxytocin is often done if delivery doesn't occur quickly). If mom or baby is in any distress, the treatment is **immediate cesarean section.** Monitoring for **DIC** and **hypotension/shock** are other important treatment measures.

More High-Yield Facts

Placenta previa is usually **painless** and is **detected** with ultrasound, while abruption is **painful** and often **not detected** by ultrasound.

In 10–20% of cases, abruption causes contained retroplacental hemorrhage (**no vaginal bleeding**—"**concealed**" abruption). However, the patient and baby will still generally have other signs/symptoms of abruption.

Case 38

Obstetrics

History

A 24-year-old, G_1P_0 woman has come to the emergency department because she is having frequent contractions. She is 40 weeks pregnant by last menstrual period and has been monitoring the timing of her contractions at home; they are now 5 minutes apart. The patient has no significant past medical history, takes no medications, and has had regular prenatal care with a normal pregnancy course. She denies the use of tobacco, alcohol, and other drugs.

Exam

T: 98.6°F   BP: 122/78   RR: 20/min.   P: 86/min.

The patient is obviously pregnant and somewhat anxious, but in no acute distress. Head and chest exams are unremarkable. Abdominal exam reveals a gravid uterus consistent with a term pregnancy. Fetal heart tones are normal. Pelvic exam shows 40% cervical effacement, and the cervix is dilated to 2 cm. The fetal head is at the level of the ischial spines. Ultrasound reveals no abnormalities, a vertex presentation, and an estimated fetal weight of 4100 grams. Maternofetal monitoring demonstrates a regular contraction pattern roughly every 5 minutes.

The woman is admitted to the labor and delivery area and her serial progress is followed (see graph of cervical dilatation and fetal descent below).

Tests

Hemoglobin: 13 g/dL (normal 12–16)
White blood cell count: 8100/μL (normal 4500–11,000)
AST: 15 u/L (normal 7–27)
Urinalysis: negative for protein, glucose, white blood cells, and bacteria
Urine drug screen: negative

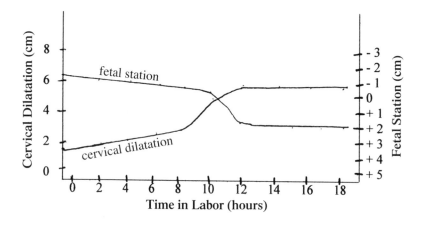

Arrested labor

Other terms are dysfunctional labor or **dystocia,** which here is likely related to fetal macrosomia (> 4000 g). The graph reveals arrest of cervical dilation and fetal descent (the straightening of both lines on the right side of the graph).

Pathophysiology

The first stage of labor starts when **regular contractions** occur **every 3–5 minutes** along **with cervical effacement and/or dilatation.** The first stage is divided into the **latent phase** (0 to 3–4 cm of dilation; irregular and slow phase) and the **active phase** (3–4 cm to full dilation; regular and fast phase). During the active phase, if the cervix dilates less than **1 cm per hour** or the fetal descent is less than **1 cm per hour,** but slower progress still occurs, a **protraction disorder** is said to present. If dilation or descent stops completely for more than **1–2 hours,** an **arrest disorder** is present. The first stage ends when the cervix is **fully dilated.** Dystocia can occur during the second stage of labor (full dilation to expulsion), which should take less than **30 minutes.**

There are multiple causes for abnormal labor progression, including **cephalopelvic disproportion (CPD),** in which the baby is too big for the birth canal (this is the **most common cause); abnormal fetal position** (e.g., **breech** presentation, transverse lie); and **ineffective uterine contractions.**

Diagnosis & Treatment

In routine deliveries, closely monitor cervical dilatation and effacement and fetal station (head position in relation to the maternal ischial spines) **every 2 hours** to check for normal progression. If protraction or arrest of labor occurs, confirm the presentation and lie of the fetus, and use physical exam and ultrasound to help determine the presence of CPD. If neither position nor CPD is the problem, **observation** is preferred for slow progress (though augmentation is commonly used), while labor **augmentation** is generally used for labor arrest.

Labor augmentation includes the use of IV **oxytocin** and **prostaglandin E$_2$ gel.** Amniotomy is *controversial.* Contraindications to labor augmentation include a **contracted maternal pelvis** (i.e., probable CPD), **prior "classic" (vertical incision) c-section, abnormal presentation or lie,** markedly preterm fetus, and acute **fetal distress.** The more *"favorable"* (e.g., effaced, dilated, and soft) the cervix, the *more likely* augmentation is to succeed. If augmentation fails or maternal/fetal distress occurs, **c-section** is indicated.

More High-Yield Facts

Oxytocin complications include uterine **hyperstimulation** (painful, ineffective contractions), uterine **rupture, water intoxication** (ADH-like effect), uterine muscle **fatigue,** and postpartum **uterine atony. Stop the infusion** if problems occur prior to delivery (half-life only 5 minutes).

Obstetrics

History

A 37-year-old, G_6P_5 woman has come to the emergency department because she is in labor, and she mentions that her "water broke." The patient is 38 weeks pregnant. Her pregnancy has gone smoothly up until this point. She is taken upstairs to the labor and delivery area after an ultrasound reveals no abnormalities and exam confirms ruptured membranes and 2 cm of cervical dilatation. The patient seems to be progressing rapidly though labor for the first few hours after admission. Suddenly, the nurse calls you and states that the woman is in respiratory distress. She was fine when you saw her 15 minutes ago.

Exam

T: 99.6°F   BP: 82/48   RR: 32/min.   P: 134/min.

The patient is in marked respiratory distress and is diaphoretic. Her skin is pale, with mottled cyanosis, and is cold and clammy to the touch. Pulses are weak and thready. Chest exam reveals a few scattered rhonchi, but the patient is unable to slow down her breathing enough to cooperate with the exam. Her heart is tachycardic with a regular rhythm. Pelvic exam reveals no obvious uterine abnormalities or hemorrhage and no change in the cervix or fetal position. Though 100% oxygen is being administered by face mask, the pulse oximetry reading is 70%. Intravenous fluids are started and stat labs are drawn. The patient's blood pressure fails to respond to fluids and she begins to convulse. She dies shortly after intubation and mechanical ventilation are started.

Tests

Hemoglobin: 11 g/dL (normal 12–16)
White blood cell count: 10,100/μL (normal 4500–11,000)
Platelets: 90,000/μL (normal 150,000–400,000)
Peripheral smear: 3+ schistocytes; normal-appearing squamous cells
D-dimer: positive
Fibrinogen: 2 μM/L (normal 4–10)
Fibrinogen split products: strongly positive
Prothrombin time (PT): 19 seconds (normal 10–14 seconds)
Partial thromboplastin time (PTT): 45 seconds (normal 25–38)
Urine drug screen: negative

Pathophysiology

Amniotic fluid embolism occurs when amniotic fluid and other intrauterine fetal debris (hair, sloughed epithelial cells) are introduced into the **maternal circulation,** generally via the uterine or placental veins. Like a venous thrombus, this material can travel into the pulmonary arterial tree. In addition to physically blocking pulmonary circulation, the amniotic fluid and debris can cause an intense **inflammatory response** and **coagulopathy** (disseminated intravascular coagulation [DIC]). Mortality is estimated at **80–90%.** Though this condition is rare, thromboembolic phenomena are a **leading cause of maternal mortality** (along with pregnancy-induced hypertension/eclampsia).

Risk factors include **placental abruption** or **uterine rupture,** increasing maternal **age,** tumultuous labor, use of **uterine stimulants** (e.g., oxytocin), **multiparity,** and intrauterine **fetal death.** This condition can occur after an abortion or before, during, or after vaginal or c-section delivery.

Diagnosis & Treatment

An amniotic fluid embolus usually presents as a **sudden, unexpected** catastrophic event. Patients may have one or more risk factors discussed above. They generally experience **sudden shortness of breath,** often without chest pain. Lightheadedness or **altered mental status** may develop.

Exam reveals **hypoxia, tachypnea, tachycardia,** and **hypotension**—all of which usually leads to **cold, clammy, and pale** skin, with mottled **cyanosis** and **diaphoresis.** A weak, thready pulse is typically present. Patients may develop **syncope, convulsions,** and/or **bleeding** from DIC. Signs of right heart failure (from acute increase in pulmonary arterial pressure) may be seen. Chest x-ray may show **pulmonary edema.** Labs may show **DIC** (decreased platelets and fibrinogen, prolonged PT and PTT, **schistocytes**/fragmented red blood cells on peripheral smear, positive D-dimer and fibrinogen split products). The diagnosis is clinical (or made at autopsy). **Fetal squamous cells** may be seen in a maternal blood sample.

Treatment is **supportive.** Oxygen (intubation and mechanical ventilation may be needed), intravenous fluids, blood products, and management of heart failure and/or convulsions may be needed.

More High-Yield Facts

Watch for DIC and/or amniotic fluid embolism after a **missed abortion** (retained dead fetus for several weeks).

Obstetrics

History

A 26-year-old, G_1P_0 woman, who is 36 weeks pregnant by last menstrual period, is experiencing uterine contractions. She says they are occurring every 5 minutes. The patient has had no regular prenatal care, but reports no problems with the pregnancy and denies any vaginal bleeding or discharge. She has no significant past medical history and takes no regular medications. The patient denies the use of tobacco, alcohol, and illicit drugs.

Exam

T: 98.6°F   BP: 118/78   RR: 16/min.   P: 84/min.

The patient is obviously pregnant and in no acute distress. Her chest is clear to auscultation. Abdominal exam reveals a gravid uterus consistent with the menstrual age. The fetal head is palpated in the uterine fundus, and the fetal heart rate is normal. Pelvic exam reveals that the cervix is dilated to 3 cm and 60% effaced. You are able to palpate the fetal buttocks and sacrum as the presenting part, but no feet are palpable. Ultrasound exam reveals no fetal anomalies and an estimated fetal weight of 3400 grams. Of the examples (see figures), which condition is described above? What is it called? How should you manage it?

Tests

Hemoglobin: 13 g/dL (normal 12–16)
White blood cell count: 7100/μL (normal 4500–11,000)
Platelets: 190,000/μL (normal 150,000–400,000)
Urinalysis: negative for protein, glucose, bacteria, and white blood cells
Urine drug screen: negative

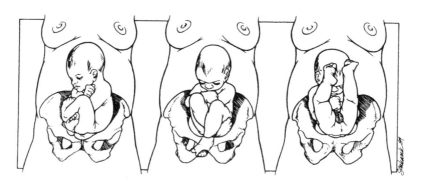

From Gabbe SG, Niebyl JR, Simpson JL (eds): Obstetrics: Normal & Problem Pregnancies. New York, Churchill Livingstone, 1986, p 465; with permission.

Breech presentation

This is a type of fetal malpresentation. The figures show, from left to right, a complete, incomplete (**footling**), and frank breech (the type this case describes).

Pathophysiology

Any presentation other than **head first** with the head **flexed (vertex)** is considered abnormal. Breech presentation is present in one-third of pregnancies in the **second trimester,** but most **spontaneously convert** to head-first position by term (**3–4%** incidence at term). **Frank (flexed thighs, extended knees)** is the most common breech (65% of cases), with **complete (flexed thighs, flexed knees)** and **incomplete (one or both legs extended below the buttocks)** less common. Risk is increased by **multiple gestation, uterine anomalies or masses, oligo/polyhydramnios,** and **fetal anomalies** and **disorders** (especially anencephaly and hydrocephalus)

Other presentations include **face** (head first in hyperextension) and **brow** (head first, neither extended nor flexed), which both often convert to vertex and can then delivery vaginally. **Shoulder** presentation mandates c-section.

Diagnosis & Treatment

Palpation (i.e., Leopold's maneuvers) reveals the fetal head in the uterine **fundus.** The type of breech can usually be determined on pelvic exam. With a frank breech, the "breech" (**buttocks, sacrum, ischial spines**) can be palpated (the only palpable part). With a complete breech, **one or both feet** can be palpated *alongside* the buttocks, which are also palpable. With an incomplete breech, **one or both feet** are palpated *alone.* **Ultrasound** is done in **all cases** to help confirm findings, estimate fetal size, and rule out fetal anomalies.

Initial management after a normal ultrasound if the baby is **at least 37 weeks** is usually **external version,** or physical fetal manipulation to convert the baby to a vertex presentation (works 50–75% of time). Conservative management is **c-section** for all breech presentations that fail version, to reduce the risk of fetal morbidity and mortality (which is increased and most commonly from anomalies, hypoxia, birth injury, and prematurity). However, a trial of vaginal delivery is acceptable in frank or complete breech (*not* incomplete breech, however) if mom is **term** with a **normal baby size** and no complicating factors.

More High-Yield Facts

On Step 2, if asked, **perform a c-section for any breech presentation.** Try external version first if given the option and the baby is term, as long as nothing else is going on (e.g., placenta previa, fetal distress).

Case 41

Obstetrics

History

A 32-year-old, G_7P_6 woman, who is 40 weeks pregnant by last menstrual period, presents with uterine contractions. She says they are occurring every 10 minutes. The patient had regular prenatal care, and no problems with the pregnancy were identified. The woman has not experienced vaginal bleeding, pain, or discharge. She has no significant past medical history and takes no regular medications. The patient denies the use of tobacco, alcohol, or illicit drugs.

Exam

T: 98.6°F   BP: 126/84   RR: 18/min.   P: 88/min.

The patient's chest is clear to auscultation. Abdominal exam reveals a gravid uterus consistent with a term gestation. The fetal heart rate is normal. Pelvic exam shows that the cervix is dilated to 2 cm and 50% effaced. Ultrasound demonstrates no abnormalities and an estimated fetal weight of 4250 grams.

The patient has a protracted course of labor and requires oxytocin for a prolonged period to augment labor. She eventually delivers a normal infant in no distress, but has roughly 1 liter of steady vaginal blood loss after delivery. No genital tract trauma or lacerations can be identified. The uterine fundus is palpable at the umbilicus and is quite boggy in consistency.

Tests

Hemoglobin: 11 g/dL (normal 12–16)
White blood cell count: 7100/μL (normal 4500–11,000)
Platelets: 290,000/μL (normal 150,000–400,000)
Prothrombin time: 11 seconds (normal 10–14)
Partial thromboplastin time: 25 seconds (normal 25–38)
Urinalysis: negative for protein, glucose, bacteria, and white blood cells
Urine drug screen: negative

Postpartum hemorrhage secondary to uterine atony

Pathophysiology

Blood loss **> 500 cc** after vaginal delivery or **> 1 liter** after c-section defines postpartum hemorrhage. The **most common cause (75% of cases) is uterine atony.** Other causes include **genital tract trauma, retained placental tissue** (the spectrum of **placenta accreta,** when placental tissue grows into the myometrium), **low placental implantation, coagulation disorders,** and **uterine inversion.**

Normally, the uterus contracts to stop hemorrhage from placental vessels after placental detachment. Uterine atony occurs when the uterine musculature **lacks the needed tone** to contract appropriately. Risk factors include **overdistension** of the uterus (**multiple gestation, large baby, polyhydramnios**), **prolonged** or **very short labor duration,** use of **oxytocin** or **magnesium** sulfate, **grandmultiparity** (parity of five or more), and **chorioamnionitis.**

Diagnosis & Treatment

In the setting of postpartum hemorrhage, standard supportive care—such as IV fluid and/or blood, placement of a Foley catheter to drain the bladder and monitor urine output, and oxygen—is given while searching for the cause. If the uterus feels **boggy,** atony is the likely cause. Examine the genital tract for lacerations and **perform repair** if found. Uterine inversion is obvious upon uterine palpation, or the inverted uterus may be **visible at the introitus.** If the placenta does not deliver or **pieces are missing** when the placenta is examined, retained placental tissue is the likely cause of hemorrhage.

Uterine atony management is **manual uterine massage** and **oxytocin. Methylergonovine** can be tried next if this fails. The last resort is **prostaglandin $F_{2\text{-alpha}}$.** If these fail to stop the bleeding, **surgery** is needed, with ligation of the **uterine** and/or **iliac arteries** and possibly hysterectomy. Uterine inversion requires **manual return** of the uterus to its normal position, often under general anesthesia and tocolysis to relax the uterus. If retained placenta/placental tissue is the cause, **manual removal** of the placenta is required with uterine **curettage** afterwards. Extensive or deep forms of placenta accreta often require **hysterectomy** to stop the bleeding. Coagulation disorders can be found during the history or with **coagulation studies** (which should be ordered in any case of hemorrhage).

More High-Yield Facts

A common cause of uterine inversion is **iatrogenic.** Don't pull hard on the umbilical cord or press on the fundus if the placenta doesn't deliver right away. Patience and gentle traction are all that is needed in most cases.

Case 42

Obstetrics

History

A 27-year-old, G_1P_1 woman seeks medical advice for "feeling lousy" and inability to breast-feed. A midwife delivered her baby at home 2 weeks earlier, and the patient had excessive postpartum hemorrhage and shock. Hospitalization and intensive care were required for both her and the baby. The patient received multiple blood transfusions, recovered a few days later, and went home. The baby is now doing fine. However, the mother says that there didn't seem to be any milk in her breasts when she got home from the hospital. She also mentions that she always feels fatigued and weak, though she denies feeling "down" or depressed, and asks when she can expect to begin menstruating again. She takes no medications and has no significant past medical history.

Exam

T: 98.6°F   BP: 116/76   RR: 14/min.   P: 74/min.

The patient is in no acute distress. Her chest is clear to auscultation, and no heart murmurs are appreciated. The woman's breasts have involuted to near their pregestational size, and no milk can be expressed from them. Abdominal and pelvic exams are unremarkable.

Tests

Hemoglobin: 12 g/dL (normal 12–16)
White blood cell count: 7100/μL (normal 4500–11,000)
Platelets: 290,000/μL (normal 150,000–400,000)
Prolactin level: undetectable (normal 2–15 ng/mL)
Thyroid stimulating hormone (TSH): 0.4 μU/mL (normal 0.5–5)
Urinalysis: negative for protein, glucose, bacteria, and white blood cells
Urine drug screen: negative

Sheehan's syndrome

Sheehan's syndrome, though rare, is a classic boards topic.

Pathophysiology

In cases of massive maternal hemorrhage or shock, **pituitary hypoxia** and **necrosis** can occur. Pituitary damage in the setting of generalized hypotension/shock is fairly clinically unique to **pregnancy,** though a late presentation (up to 10 years after the causative incident) can impede the diagnosis.

Posterior pituitary function is often **spared** (though diabetes insipidus has been reported from Sheehan's syndrome), but varying degrees of anterior pituitary function are lost. In *all* cases, prolactin secretion is lost, resulting in the inability to breast-feed. The sex hormones (LH and FSH), growth hormone, and thyroid (TSH) and adrenocortical function (ACTH) can all be affected.

Diagnosis & Treatment

The boards will always give you a history of **severe pregnancy-related hemorrhage,** which will often include the mention of **shock** and/or **multiple transfusions.** Most often, patients present with **inability to breast-feed** and **rapid breast involution** early in the postpartum period. Vague constitutional symptoms are also common, such as **nausea, weakness,** and **fatigue.** However, if a woman chooses to **bottle-feed** her baby, she may not notice any symptoms for **months or years.** Though menstruation usually returns within 6–8 weeks after delivery in the absence of breast-feeding, women with Sheehan's syndrome have **persistent amenorrhea** after delivery.

Clinical symptoms from hypothyroidism, hypoadrenalism, or infertility usually take **months or even several years** to develop or be noticed. Clues to these endocrine abnormalities are the classic symptoms/signs and lab results.

Diagnosis is made with the right history in the presence of appropriate laboratory changes (low prolactin, TSH, ACTH, LH, FSH and/or GH). A **pituitary neoplasm** or other lesion must be excluded, generally with an **MRI** of the brain. Treatment is **hormone replacement,** including estrogen, thyroid hormone, and corticosteroids.

More High-Yield Facts

On the boards, more than one pituitary-related endocrine abnormality with a history of pregnancy-related hemorrhage and *no* bitemporal hemianopsia = Sheehan's syndrome.

Case 43

Obstetrics

History

A 17-year-old, G_1P_0 woman is experiencing uterine contractions. She is 30 weeks pregnant by last menstrual period and an ultrasound performed in the first trimester. The patient says her contractions are regular and are occurring every 10 minutes. She denies vaginal bleeding or discharge, and routine prenatal care has revealed no problems in the pregnancy up to this point. Her past medical history is unremarkable, and the woman takes no medications. She does not use alcohol or drugs, but smokes about one-half pack of cigarettes per day.

Exam

T: 98.7°F   BP: 118/76   RR: 16/min.   P: 84/min.

The patient is in no acute distress. Her chest is clear to auscultation, and no heart murmurs are appreciated. Abdominal examination reveals a gravid uterus consistent with a 30-week pregnancy. Fetal heart tones are normal. There is no discharge or evidence of ruptured membranes on pelvic exam. The cervix is dilated 1 cm and 20% effaced.

Maternofetal monitoring demonstrates regular, coordinated contractions every 10 minutes and a reassuring fetal heart strip. Ultrasound shows no abnormalities and a fetal size consistent with 30 weeks gestational age.

Tests

Hemoglobin: 12 g/dL (normal 12–16)
White blood cell count: 7100/μL (normal 4500–11,000)
Platelets: 290,000/μL (normal 150,000–400,000)
Urinalysis: negative for protein, glucose, bacteria, and white blood cells
Sodium: 140 meq/L (normal 135–145)
Potassium: 4.2 meq/L (normal 3.5–5)
Creatinine: 0.6 mg/dL (normal 0.6–1.5)
BUN: 8 mg/dL (normal 8–25)
Urine drug screen: negative

Pathophysiology

Preterm labor is "true labor" that occurs **between 20 and 37 weeks** (some use a fetal weight between 500–2500 grams instead). True labor means regular contractions with cervical changes. Preterm births are estimated to occur in **5–10%** of all pregnancies in the U.S.

Numerous risk factors include **prior preterm delivery** or miscarriage, **smoking, low** socioeconomic status, congenital fetal or maternal uterine **anomalies,** extremes of reproductive **age, infections** (especially urinary tract or pelvic), **multiple gestation,** and poor nutritional status. Preterm labor and delivery markedly increases the incidence of **perinatal morbidity and mortality,** primarily from complications of **prematurity.**

Diagnosis & Treatment

Women present with uterine **contractions** in the third trimester prior to 37 weeks. Risk factors discussed above may be present. Initial assessment includes determining whether or not the **membranes have ruptured,** the status of the cervix, and uterine contraction frequency. **Ultrasound** is done to evaluate the fetus and rule out other problems (e.g., placenta previa).

Once preterm labor is confirmed, initial management consists of **bed rest** and **hydration.** These measures alone will stop contractions in some women. Any **correctable risk factors** are also addressed (e.g., treatment of a urinary tract infection with antibiotics, smoking cessation). If these measures fail, **tocolytic therapy** (stops uterine contractions), usually with **beta-2 agonists** (e.g., ritodrine, terbutaline), is often advised. **Contraindications** to tocolysis include maternal or fetal **distress,** pre-eclampsia, severe fetal anomalies, and chorioamnionitis.

The point of tocolytic therapy is to **delay delivery** at least until 48 hours of **corticosteroids** (e.g., betamethasone) can be given to **hasten fetal lung maturity** and prevent respiratory distress in the newborn. Usually, **amniocentesis** is performed and the amniotic fluid is assessed for lecithin (L), sphingomyelin (S), and phosphatidyl-glycerol (PG). An **L:S ratio greater than 2:1** and/or the **presence of PG** are good predictors of fetal lung maturity. If these values do not support mature fetal lungs, steroids are given—as long as prolonged membrane rupture is not present (increased infection risk, less benefit). If it works, tocolysis can be used until **term.**

More High-Yield Facts

Beta-2 agonist side-effects include **tachycardia, blood pressure** changes, chest pain, **pulmonary edema,** and hyperglycemia. **Magnesium** therapy is an option in those with heart disease or intolerance of beta-2 agonists.

Case 44

Obstetrics

History

A 27-year-old, G_3P_0 woman has suffered three successive spontaneous miscarriages, the most recent occurring 5 weeks ago. Each of the pregnancies ended before the end of the first term. She and her husband are frustrated and want to know why this keeps happening. The woman has no known medical problems and takes no regular medications. She does not smoke, drink alcohol, or use illicit drugs. There is no family history of genetic disorders as far as the patient knows, either in her or her husband's family.

Exam

T: 98.8°F   BP: 120/78   RR: 14/min.   P: 84/min.

The patient is healthy appearing, and no skin rashes are identified. Head, neck, chest, and abdominal exams reveal no abnormalities. There are no uterine or adnexal abnormalities apparent on pelvic exam. Speculum exam demonstrates a normal-appearing cervix and vagina, with no discharge identified. External genitalia and overall sexual development are normal.

Tests

Hemoglobin: 13 g/dL (normal 12–16)
White blood cell count: 8100/µL (normal 4500–11,000)
Platelets: 310,000/µL (normal 150,000–400,000)
Sodium: 139 meq/L (normal 135–145)
Potassium: 4 meq/L (normal 3.5–5)
Creatinine: 0.8 mg/dL (normal 0.6–1.5)
BUN: 10 mg/dL (normal 8–25)
Glucose: 78 mg/dL (normal fasting: 70–110)
Thyroid stimulating hormone: 2.2 µU/mL (normal 0.5–5)
Antinuclear antibody: negative
Anti-phospholipid antibody: negative
Urinalysis: negative for protein, glucose, bacteria, and white blood cells
Urine drug screen: negative
Cervical cultures: pending

Recurrent miscarriage

Pathophysiology

The classic definition of recurrent miscarriage is **three successive** spontaneous abortions. It is estimated that up to **15%** of clinically recognizable pregnancies end in miscarriage, and no reason can be found in the majority of cases. However, when repeated miscarriages occur, the likelihood of an **identifiable cause** increases dramatically. Investigation of these causes is usually recommended after two successive first-trimester losses or a single second-trimester miscarriage.

Diagnosis & Treatment

Women who **smoke** or **drink alcohol** during pregnancy have an increased risk of miscarriage. **Hypothyroidism, systemic lupus erythematosus,** and **diabetes mellitus** are medical conditions that must be excluded with testing. The **antiphospholipid antibody syndrome** (**prolonged PTT** value though patients have an increased risk of thrombosis) and **anticardiolipin** antibodies (cause a **false-positive VDRL syphilis test**) are other autoimmune disorders that can be tested for directly. Genetic testing can detect maternal or paternal **chromosomal disorders.**

Uterine abnormalities that may cause recurrent abortion include **cervical incompetence, congenital** uterine **anomalies, fibroids,** and **intrauterine adhesions** (usually from prior **dilatation and curettage**). These uterine abnormalities can generally be detected with a **hysterosalpingogram** (contrast is injected into the uterus and x-rays are taken). Rarely, recurrent abortions can be caused by *Mycoplasma, Listeria,* or *Toxoplasma* infections.

After the above conditions are tested for, treatment is directed at any abnormalities found (**50%** of cases remain **idiopathic** even after the work-up). **Psychological support** and counseling are important adjunctive therapies, as miscarriages can be devastating to the patient and her family.

More High-Yield Facts

Recurrent, painless, and rapid miscarriages in the **second trimester** are classically due to cervical incompetence. A wide cervical os is often present on exam. Treatment is placement of a **cervical suture (cerclage)** at **14–16 weeks,** which can be removed at term. Intrauterine exposure to **diethylstilbestrol** is a classic risk factor for cervical incompetence.

The antiphospholipid antibody syndrome can also cause **thrombocytopenia** and **early pre-eclampsia.** Treatment with **aspirin** plus either **prednisone** or **heparin** reduces miscarriage rates as well as the risk of thrombosis. Lupus may or may not be present.

Case 45

Obstetrics

History

A 27-year-old, G_2P_1 woman presents for her first prenatal visit after a home pregnancy test turned out to be positive. Her last menstrual period was 8 weeks ago. The patient had no prenatal care during her first pregnancy, but claims there were no problems with the pregnancy until delivery. The woman ended up needing a cesarean section because her baby was "too big to pass vaginally." The baby weighed 10 pounds, 3 ounces (4560 grams) at birth after 8.5 months gestation, according to the patient.

The patient's past medical history is significant only for obesity. She does not smoke, drink alcohol, or use drugs. Family history is notable for diabetes in both the patient's parents and two of her brothers.

Exam

T: 98.8°F   BP: 120/78   RR: 14/min.   P: 84/min.

The patient is obese, but in no acute distress. Head, chest, and abdominal exams are unremarkable. Pelvic exam reveals a mildly enlarged, smooth, somewhat globular uterus consistent with early pregnancy. No adnexal masses are noted. No abnormalities are found on speculum and external genitalia exams.

Tests

Hemoglobin: 13 g/dL (normal 12–16)
White blood cell count: 8100/μL (normal 4500–11,000)
Platelets: 310,000/μL (normal 150,000–400,000)
Sodium: 139 meq/L (normal 135–145)
Potassium: 4 meq/L (normal 3.5–5)
Creatinine: 0.8 mg/dL (normal 0.6–1.5)
BUN: 10 mg/dL (normal 8–25)
Glucose, fasting: 115 mg/dL (normal fasting 70–110)
Urinalysis: negative for protein, bacteria, and white blood cells; trace glucose
β-hCG, qualitative: positive

Pathophysiology

Diabetes can be pre-existing or pregnancy can result in "gestational" diabetes (GD), which begins during pregnancy and ends shortly after delivery. There is an increased risk of developing diabetes during pregnancy because of hormonal changes that favor hyperglycemia. GD is the **most common medical complication of pregnancy.**

Maternal complications of GD include polyhydramnios, **pre-eclampsia,** and an increased rate of **c-sections** and infections. Fetal complications include **macrosomia, birth trauma, neonatal hypoglycemia, stillbirth,** and **delayed organ maturity** (e.g., increased risk of respiratory distress syndrome). Congenital **anomalies** (especially cardiovascular, caudal regression, and neural tube defects) are caused by pre-existing diabetes, as GD usually begins *after* the organs have formed. **GD increases the risk for future maternal DM** as well as **obesity and DM in the child.**

Risk factors for maternal diabetes include **age > 25; obesity; family history** of DM; and a history of a prior **macrosomic infant** (> 4000 grams), **polyhydramnios,** stillbirth, or **recurrent spontaneous abortions.**

Diagnosis & Treatment

All non-diabetic women should be screened at **24–28 weeks'** gestation—the period when insulin resistance is peaking. If risk factors for GD are present, also screen at the **first prenatal visit.** Screening is done with a plasma glucose level drawn 1–2 hours after an oral glucose load (glucose "**challenge**" test). If the level is ≥ **140 mg/dl,** the patient is given the **gold standard** test for GD: a 3-hour, 100-g oral glucose "**tolerance**" test (**OGTT**) after an overnight fast. In the OGTT, the patient's glucose levels are measured before the oral load (> 105 mg/dL abnormal) and 1 hour (> 190 abnormal), 2 hours (> 165 abnormal), and 3 hours (> 145 abnormal) later. **Two or more abnormal values** gives a diagnosis of GD.

Treatment includes **diet, exercise,** and **insulin** if needed. Oral hypoglycemic agents are *contraindicated,* as they cross the placenta. Frequent blood monitoring and insulin dose adjustments are used to reduce the risk of complications. The better the glucose control, the better the outcome. Prenatal **ultrasound** and **biophysical profile testing** near term are done routinely due to the increased risks GD introduces to a pregnancy.

More High-Yield Facts

Fetal macrosomia is due to maternal GD *"until proven otherwise."*

Obstetrics

History

A 37-year-old, G_4P_3 woman is in your office for a routine prenatal visit. She is at 17 weeks' gestation by last menstrual period. She has no complaints and has three healthy children, all delivered vaginally. The patient inquires about screening for Down syndrome, which a friend told her is more common in older women. She asks to be tested. The patient's past medical and family histories are unremarkable, and her only medication is a daily multivitamin.

Exam

T: 98.5°F   BP: 126/82   RR: 16/min.   P: 80/min.

The patient is healthy appearing. Head, chest, and abdominal exams are unremarkable. The uterine size is consistent with a 17-week gestation. Fetal heart tones are normal. No adnexal masses are appreciated. Speculum and external genitalia exams reveal no abnormalities.

Tests

Hemoglobin: 14 g/dL (normal 12–16)
White blood cell count: 6600/μL (normal 4500–11,000)
Platelets: 280,000/μL (normal 150,000–400,000)
Creatinine: 0.9 mg/dL (normal 0.6–1.5)
Glucose, fasting: 85 mg/dL (normal fasting 70–110)
Urinalysis: negative for protein, glucose, bacteria. and white blood cells
Alpha-fetoprotein: low for dates
Unconjugated estriol: low for dates
Human chorionic gonadotropin: high for dates

Pathophysiology

Certain fetal anomalies (e.g., Down syndrome, **neural tube defects**) can often be detected using **maternal serum alpha-fetoprotein (AFP) level** screening. When compared to a chart of "normal values" for a given gestational age, abnormal values of AFP markedly **increase the risk** of these fetal anomalies. The addition of maternal serum unconjugated **estriol** and **human chorionic gonadotropin (hCG)** levels has increased the detection rate for **Down syndrome.** These three tests are called the "triple screen." Presently, additional Down markers are also being used (e.g., "quadruple screen" by adding an **inhibin** level, screening **ultrasound** to detect specific Down anomalies).

Diagnosis & Treatment

Screening for Down syndrome and neural tube defects (e.g., **anencephaly, spina bifida**) is offered to all women and is performed at **15–20 weeks.** It is strongly advised for women **over age 35,** as the risk of chromosomal disorders (e.g., Down syndrome) is markedly increased. An **elevated AFP** may indicate **inaccurate dates** (**most common** cause), **multiple gestation, fetal demise,** a **neural tube defect,** or a **ventral wall defect** (e.g., **omphalocele, gastroschisis**). A **low AFP** may indicate **inaccurate dates** (**most common** cause), **fetal demise, Down syndrome,** or **trisomy 18.** Memorizing the other markers is probably not worth the effort, but Down syndrome causes low estriol and high hCG.

If the AFP value is abnormal, perform an **ultrasound** to rule out inaccurate dates, fetal demise, and multiple gestation, as well as to look for any physical anomalies. If the ultrasound does not reveal the cause of the abnormal AFP, recommend **amniocentesis** (at **16–20 weeks**). The amniotic fluid **AFP level** and **acetyl-cholinesterase level** (a specific marker that is present with neural tube defects) are measured, and a **fetal karyotype** is performed (detects Down syndrome and trisomy 18).

Genetic and psychological **counseling** can then be given based on the results of these tests. The majority of positive tests end up being **false positives,** so reassure your patients to reduce anxiety.

More High-Yield Facts

Chorionic villus sampling can also be used to detect specific genetic abnormalities in those with a **family history** or **previously affected child.** This test can be done at **9–12 weeks** (earlier than amniocentesis), but it *cannot* detect neural tube or ventral wall defects (can't measure AFP, can only check for chromosomal/genetic disorders). The procedure carries a **1% risk of miscarriage** (higher than amniocentesis), but allows for a first-trimester abortion if positive.

Case 47

Obstetrics

History

A 35-year-old, G_8P_7 woman presents at 42 weeks' gestation (by last menstrual period) claiming to be in labor. She estimates her contractions to be 8–10 minutes apart. She had no routine prenatal care, but has had no problems with the pregnancy. The patient has seven healthy children, five of whom were delivered by cesarean section. Past medical history is insignificant, and she takes no regular medications. She denies the use of tobacco, alcohol, and illicit drugs.

Exam

T: 98.5°F   BP: 128/84   RR: 16/min.   P: 86/min.

The patient is obviously pregnant and in no acute distress between contractions. Head and chest exams are unremarkable. Abdominal exam reveals a smooth, gravid uterus consistent with a term pregnancy. Cervical exam shows 3 cm of cervical dilatation, 60% effacement, and a +1 fetal station.

The woman insists on delivering the child vaginally and is admitted to the labor and delivery area. Ultrasound demonstrates no abnormalities and an estimated fetal size of 4300 grams. After 2 hours of slow progression, the woman suddenly cries out in pain, saying that it feels like someone stabbed her in the lower abdomen. You discover alteration of the abdominal contour and retraction of the fetal head higher than its previous level. A blood pressure check reveals severe hypotension, and the woman develops altered mental status. A non-reassuring fetal heart rate pattern is noted on the monitor.

Tests

Hemoglobin: 12 g/dL (normal 12–16)
White blood cell count: 6600/μL (normal 4500–11,000)
Platelets: 280,000/μL (normal 150,000–400,000)
Creatinine: 0.9 mg/dL (normal 0.6–1.5)
Urinalysis: negative for protein, glucose, bacteria, and white blood cells

Pathophysiology

Complete **full-thickness** rupture through the uterine musculature is an **obstetric emergency** that requires prompt diagnosis and treatment. Partial rupture (**dehiscence**) is often asymptomatic and of little clinical consequence. Uterine rupture can be seen **before** or **during labor.** Risk factors include **prior uterine surgery** (e.g., c-section, myomectomy for fibroids), **oxytocin** use, **grand multiparity** (five or more deliveries), **uterine distension** (e.g., polyhydramnios, fetal macrosomia), **dystocia/difficult delivery, trauma,** and **abnormal fetal lie.**

Diagnosis & Treatment

The classic patient has one or more risk factors described above and develops **sudden, severe abdominal pain** near term (either spontaneously or after abdominal trauma). **Vaginal bleeding** can be heavy, mild, *or absent,* but fairly heavy bleeding into the peritoneal cavity is typical *whether or not* vaginal bleeding is present.

Physical exam classically reveals an **abnormal abdominal or uterine contour** (most obvious when it occurs in the setting of serial examinations), and **fetal parts may be discretely palpable** if they protrude through the rupture into the peritoneal cavity. The presenting fetal part may **retract** back up into the birth canal as well. Patients can rapidly develop **hypotension, tachycardia, altered mental status,** and **shock.**

Treatment in this setting is **immediate laparotomy** to deliver the baby, stop the hemorrhage, and repair the uterus. Shock management is also required.

More High-Yield Facts

After a "**modern**" c-section (**low, transverse uterine incision**), an attempt at future vaginal delivery is **allowed** and generally **encouraged,** as the risk of rupture is **low** (around 0.5%). However, after a "**classical**" c-section (**vertical uterine incision,** often extending above the lower uterine segment) or other type of c-section incision, future vaginal delivery is **contraindicated** due to the **increased risk** (around 5%) of uterine rupture. **Elective c-section** is generally scheduled before labor starts in these cases.

Sudden hypotension and shock without visible external hemorrhage is generally due to uterine rupture, **uterine inversion,** or **amniotic fluid (AF) embolus.** On the boards, physical findings and/or history will be given to help you diagnose inversion or rupture. AF embolus usually causes no specific findings (just shock), so is likely if no other findings are present.

Case 48

Obstetrics

History

A 24-year-old, G_1P_1 woman is in the hospital on postpartum day 3 after a cesarean section. She complains of chills and mild lower abdominal pain that has been getting steadily worse since yesterday afternoon and is unrelated to her surgical incision. The patient initially presented in active labor with ruptured membranes, but needed a c-section after a prolonged labor due to failure to progress. The child is currently doing well in the neonatal nursery, and the patient has been breast-feeding and ambulating successfully.

Exam

T: 101.3°F   BP: 120/76   RR: 16/min.   P: 82/min.

Physical exam reveals slight scleral pallor; no skin rashes are identified. The patient's chest is clear to auscultation. Breast exam indicates no abnormalities or tenderness. Abdominal exam demonstrates normal bowel sounds and a clean, dry c-section incision. The uterus is quite tender on palpation. No adnexal masses are noted. Speculum exam reveals somewhat purulent and foul-smelling lochia. No lacerations or lesions are identified.

Tests

Hemoglobin: 12 g/dL (normal 12–16)
White blood cell count: 12,600/µL (normal 4500–11,000)
Platelets: 330,000/µL (normal 150,000–400,000)
Creatinine: 0.9 mg/dL (normal 0.6–1.5)
Urinalysis: negative for protein, glucose, bacteria, and white blood cells
Chest x-ray: no abnormalities

Endometritis (endomyometritis)

Pathophysiology

Endometritis is infection of the lining of the uterus and the adjacent myometrium. It is a **common cause of postpartum fever.** The infection is usually **polymicrobial,** and anaerobes are present in the majority of cases. It can progress to involve tissue adjacent to the uterus (known as **parametritis** or pelvic cellulitis) and can lead to pelvic peritonitis, abscess formation, septic pelvic thrombophlebitis, and **septic shock.**

Risk factors for endometritis include **premature** or **prolonged** rupture of the membranes, **prolonged labor, frequent vaginal examinations** during labor, **cesarean section** delivery, **retained placental fragments**/manual removal of the placenta, anemia, cervical/vaginal lacerations, and poor hygiene.

Diagnosis & Treatment

Endometritis presents with a temperature **> 100.4°F or 38 °C** for 2 or more consecutive days after delivery, starting within 10 days postpartum, classically starting **2–3 days** after delivery. Patients classically have **lower abdominal pain or discomfort** and foul-smelling or purulent lochia.

Exam reveals **fever, foul-smelling** and/or **purulent lochial discharge,** and **uterine tenderness.** Obtain anaerobic and aerobic **cultures** of the **blood, cervix,** and **uterine cavity** before starting antibiotics. Generally, you should also obtain urine cultures. Subsequently, give **broad-spectrum antibiotics** (e.g., ampicillin sulbactam or cefoxitin plus doxycycline) to cover **anaerobes** and *Chlamydia;* improvement is usually seen in 2–4 days.

If improvement doesn't occur by 4–7 days (especially in the case of continued high, spiking fevers), a **pelvic abscess** or **septic pelvic thrombophlebitis** may have developed. A **CT scan** can detect an abscess, which will need surgical or catheter **drainage.** If no abscess is seen, give **heparin** for presumed septic pelvic thrombophlebitis; the fever should resolve and symptoms improve **within 2–3 days** of starting heparin therapy.

More High-Yield Facts

The other common causes of postpartum fever include **breast engorgement, mastitis, atelectasis, wound infection, urinary tract infection,** and **deep venous thrombosis.**

Frequent hand-washing and limiting the number of vaginal exams during labor are easy ways to reduce the risk of endometritis.

Case 49

Obstetrics

History

A 28-year-old, G_1P_0, pregnant woman comes to the emergency department complaining of fever and lower abdominal pain. She is 34 weeks pregnant. The patient mentions that she had sudden onset of a fairly heavy, clear, watery vaginal discharge 4 days ago that has gotten much better since. She denies contractions or vaginal bleeding, and states that the pregnancy has been problem free, despite lack of prenatal care.

Exam

T: 101.7°F   BP: 118/80   RR: 16/min.   P: 98/min.

The patient appears unkempt and acutely ill. Head and chest exams are unremarkable. Abdominal exam reveals a gravid uterus of appropriate size that is tender to palpation. Fetal heart tones demonstrate tachycardia. No rebound tenderness or guarding is present, and bowel sounds are normal. Speculum exam shows a thick, purulent, yellowish discharge, and the cervix appears to be closed.

In addition, there is some clear fluid pooled in the posterior vaginal fornix. This fluid is applied to a glass slide and allowed to dry, for microscopic viewing (see figure). Application of the fluid to a piece of nitrazine paper causes the paper to change from yellow to blue. Ultrasound exam reveals oligohydramnios, but no other abnormalities.

Tests

Hemoglobin: 12 g/dL (normal 12–16)   WBCs: 14,600/μL
Neutrophils: 84%   Platelets: 330,000/μL
Creatinine: 0.9 mg/dL (normal 0.6–1.5)
Urinalysis: negative for protein, glucose, bacteria, and white blood cells

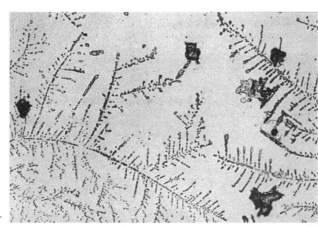

From Scott JR, et al (eds): Danforth's Obstetrics and Gynecology, 7th ed. Philadelphia, Lippincott, 1988, pp 305–315; with permission.

The present patient exhibits preterm premature rupture of the membranes (PPROM). The figure shows the classic ferning pattern of amniotic fluid.

Pathophysiology

Chorioamnionitis is an intrauterine infection of the **fetal membranes and amniotic fluid** that is usually polymicrobial and due to bacterial ascension from the lower genital tract. It is classically seen in the setting of **PROM** or **PPROM** (term or preterm membrane rupture *before* the onset of labor), as intact membranes help protect against ascending infection.

Risk factors for PPROM include **cervicitis** or **vaginitis, smoking,** prior **history** of PPROM, cervical **incompetence,** and **polyhydramnios.**

Diagnosis & Treatment

The history of ruptured membranes can range from "my water broke" to a **clear vaginal discharge.** The development of chorioamnionitis results in **fever, leukocytosis, abdominal pain** or discomfort **(uterine tenderness),** and/or a **purulent** cervical **discharge.** Take **cultures** of any discharge.

Membrane rupture is confirmed with speculum exam, which classically reveals **clear amniotic fluid pooling** in the posterior vaginal fornix. This fluid turns **nitrazine paper** from yellow to **blue** (due to its **alkaline** pH) and causes a **fern-like pattern** ("ferning") of sodium chloride crystals when dried and viewed microscopically.

Treatment of PPROM or PROM is usually observation in uncomplicated cases. Most women near term will spontaneously go into labor **within 48 hours** of membrane rupture. Close monitoring is needed to detect early infection. Some induce labor if the patient is at term and the cervix is "favorable." Treatment of chorioamnionitis is **broad-spectrum antibiotics** to cover **anaerobes** and *Chlamydia* (e.g., ampicillin sulbactam or cefoxitin plus doxycycline). The child is then delivered, either by induction of labor and vaginal delivery, or by c-section, unless significantly premature (rare).

More High-Yield Facts

Group B streptococci (GBS) are part of the normal flora in some women, but are a **common cause of chorioamnionitis and neonatal sepsis** and **meningitis. Routine screening** (using culture) **of all women** is advised at **35–37 weeks,** with intrapartum treatment given for those with positive cultures. Alternatively, women with risk factors for GBS (e.g., prolonged ruptured membranes, fever, prior GBS) can be **treated empirically** during the intrapartum period. Treatment in either case is **penicillin** or **ampicillin (clindamycin** for penicillin-allergic patients).

Obstetrics

History

A 25-year-old, G_1P_0 woman has an appointment for her first prenatal visit. The patient is 24 weeks pregnant by last menstrual period. Her pregnancy has been problem-free thus far. There is no significant past medical history, and she takes no regular medications. The patient does not smoke, drink alcohol, or use illicit drugs. She denies any history of sexually transmitted diseases.

Exam

T: 98.3°F   BP: 128/84   RR: 16/min.   P: 84/min.

The patient looks pregnant, but is in no acute distress. Her sclerae are somewhat pale. Chest exam is unremarkable. Abdominal exam reveals a gravid uterus with a fundal height of 30 cm. There are two sets of fetal heart tones noted during auscultation. Speculum exam demonstrates no abnormalities.

An ultrasound confirms the presence of twins. The patient asks you what kinds of problems she can expect because she is carrying twins.

Tests

Hemoglobin: 10 g/dL (normal 12–16)
White blood cell count: 6600/μL (normal 4500–11,000)
Creatinine: 0.9 mg/dL (normal 0.6–1.5)
Urinalysis: negative for protein, bacteria, and white blood cells; trace glucose
Fasting glucose: 94 mg/dL (normal 70–110)

This patient also has anemia.

Pathophysiology

Twins occur in roughly 1 of 90 natural pregnancies in the U.S. (they occur in 10–30% of women on fertility drugs). Multiple gestations result in **increased maternal and fetal morbidity and mortality.**

Maternal complications include **anemia,** hypertension/**pre-eclampsia,** premature labor, **polyhydramnios** (which may cause respiratory difficulty), and **postpartum hemorrhage/uterine atony.** Fetal complications include **malpresentation, placenta previa** and **abruption, premature** rupture of the membranes, **vasa previa, prematurity,** congenital anomalies, and **intrauterine growth retardation** (IUGR).

Diagnosis & Treatment

Women with twins usually have a **"size-dates" discrepancy** when the fundal height is measured. **Two sets** of fetal heart tones may also be noted. **Above-average weight gain** in mom is common and normal. In some cases, the presence of twins is not known until the time of labor and delivery, which increases the risk of **complications. Ultrasound** is an easy way to confirm the diagnosis.

Women with twins can be delivered **vaginally** if both babies have a vertex presentation (50% of cases), though some perform c-section for all twin deliveries. For all other presentations (vertex-breech, breech-vertex, or breech-breech), **cesarean section** is fairly routine. Average gestation is **35 weeks** in twins, versus **39 weeks** in singleton births.

More High-Yield Facts

Are they **monozygotic (identical)** or **dizygotic (fraternal)**? If the **sex** or **blood type** is different, they're dizygotic. If the placenta is **monochorionic,** they're monozygotic. This "poor man's" method can make the diagnosis in 80% of cases (**HLA typing** is needed for the remaining 20%).

The **twin-twin transfusion syndrome** occurs when an arteriovenous anastomosis exists in twins that share a placenta. One twin becomes a blood "donor" and develops **hypovolemia, hypotension, anemia,** and **IUGR.** The "recipient" twin develops **hypervolemia, polycythemia,** and **edema.** This syndrome is suspected when the twins have a marked **size discrepancy.**

Start close monitoring with serial **biophysical profile testing** and **ultrasound** early in the third trimester in all cases of multiple gestation because of the higher complication risk.

CASE INDEX

Notes

Notes

Notes

Notes

Notes

Notes

Notes

Notes

Notes

Notes

Notes

Notes

Notes

Notes

Notes

Notes

Notes

Notes

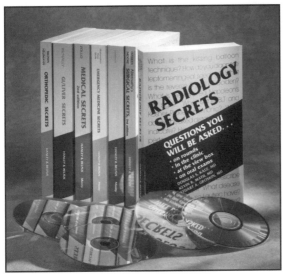

More Board Review Help

Adam Brochert, MD, is a young physician who scored in the 99th percentile on Step 2 and has extensively researched the recent administrations of the USMLE. In addition to the Platinum Vignettes™, Dr. Brochert has written these best-selling USMLE reviews.

Crush the Boards

Crammed full of information from recent administrations of Step 2, this valuable review provides these features: high-yield information in a well-written, easily accessible format; complete coverage without being overwhelming; information is presented in the form it is asked about on Step 2; all subspecialty topics covered in Step 2 are addressed; text is filled with many helpful tables and illustrations; tips, insights, and guidance are offered on how best to prepare and what to expect.
2000 • 230 pages • illustrated • ISBN 1-56053-366-8 • $28 (US), $33 (outside US)

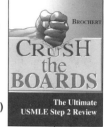

USMLE Step 2 Secrets

High-yield information taken from recent administrations of Step 2 is presented in the proven format of the best-selling Secrets Series®. Not just for memorization, Secrets presents a logical series of questions and answers that make you think about the answers and organize your thoughts. You will increase your confidence and guarantee your success on Step 2.
2000 • 265 pages • illustrated • ISBN 1-56053-451-6 • $35.95 (US), $40.95 (outside US)

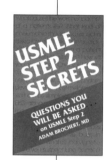

USMLE Step 2 Mock Exam

This valuable review is unique in the extent to which it simulates USMLE Step 2 conditions. Not only do the questions adhere to Step 2 clinical vignette formulations, but explanations ensure that you understand why your answer is right or wrong, a subject index allows you to focus on areas where you may need more study, and photos illustrate many of the conditions. Bottom line is that this popular review will help you master Step 2 material and increase your Step 2 scores. **USMLE STEP 2 MOCK EXAM also available in PDA format!**
2001 • 345 pages • illustrated • ISBN 1-56053-462-1 • $29 (US), $34 (outside US)

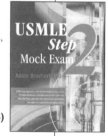

Crush Step 3

The author of the highly popular Crush the Boards presents this easy-to-use and effective high-yield review for Step 3. This review is perfect for the busy house officer who needs a review that hits all the important concepts and commonly tested topics in a concise format. The coverage also weaves in the kind of case-based scenarios that are one of the important keys to success in Step 3. It also contains the authors tips and guidance on how to prepare and what to expect. If you know the concepts in this book, you will Crush Step 3!
2001 • 225 pages • illustrated • ISBN 1-56053-484-2 • $29 (US), $34 (outside US)

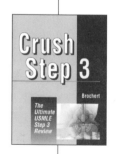

To order go to www.hanleyandbelfus.com